Histological Typing of Skin Tumours

Springer
Berlin
Heidelberg
New York
Barcelona
Budapest
Hong Kong
London
Milan
Paris
Santa Clara
Singapore
Tokyo

World Health Organization

The series *International Histological Classification of Tumours* consists of the following volumes. Each of these volumes – apart from volumes 1 and 2, which have already been revised – will appear in a revised edition within the next few years. Volumes of the current editions can be ordered through WHO, Distribution and Sales, Avenue Appia, CH-1211 Geneva 27.

1. Histological typing of lung tumours (1967, second edition 1981)
2. Histological typing of breast tumours (1968, second edition 1981)
4. Histological typing of oral and oropharyngeal tumours (1971)
8. Cytology of the female genital tract (1973)
9. Histological typing of ovarian tumours (1973)
10. Histological typing of urinary bladder tumours (1973)
12. Histological typing of skin tumours (1974)
14. Histological and cytological typing of neoplastic diseases of haematopoietic and lymphoid tissues (1976)
16. Histological typing of testis tumours (1977)
17. Cytology of non-gynaecological sites (1977)
22. Histological typing of prostate tumours (1980)
23. Histological typing of endocrine tumours (1980)
24. Histological typing of tumours of the eye and its adnexa (1980)
25. Histological typing of kidney tumours (1981)

A coded compendium of the International Histological Classification of Tumours (1978).

The following volumes have already appeared in a revised edition with Springer-Verlag:

Histological Typing of Thyroid Tumours, 2nd edn. Hedinger/Williams/Sobin (1988)

Histological Typing of Intestinal Tumours, 2nd edn. Jass/Sobin (1989)

Histological Typing of Oesophageal and Gastric Tumours, 2nd edn. Watanabel/Jass/Sobin (1990)

Histological Typing of Tumours of the Gallbladder and Extrahepatic Bile Ducts, 2nd edn. Albores-Saavedra/Henson/Sobin (1990)

Histological Typing of Tumours of the Upper Respiratory Tract and Ear, 2nd edn. Shanmugaratnam/Sobin (1981)

Histological Typing of Salivary Gland Tumours, 2nd edn. Seifert (1991)

Histological Typing of Odontogenic Tumours, 2nd edn. Kramer/Pindborg/Shear (1992)

Histological Typing of Tumours of the Central Nervous System, 2nd edn. Kleihues/Burger/Scheithauer (1993)

Histological Typing of Bone Tumours, 2nd edn. Schajowicz (1993)

Histological Typing of Soft Tissue Tumours, 2nd edn. Weiss (1994)

Histological Typing of Female Genital Tract Tumours, 2nd edn. Scully et al. (1994)

Histological Typing of Tumours of the Liver, 2nd edn. Ishak et al. (1994)

Histological Typing of Tumours of the Exocrine Pancreas, 2nd edn. Klöppel/Solcia/Longnecker/Capella/Sobin (1996)

Histological Typing of Skin Tumours, 2nd edn. Heenan/Elder/Sobin (1996)

Histological Typing of Skin Tumours

P.J. Heenan, D.E. Elder, and L.H. Sobin

In Collaboration with Pathologists in 10 Countries

Second Edition

With 143 Figures

Springer

P.J. Heenan
Associate Professor
Department of Pathology
University of Western Australia
Queen Elizabeth II Medical Center
Perth, WA 6009, Australia

D.E. Elder
Professor
Department of Pathology and Laboratory Medicine
University of Pennsylvania School of Medicine
Philadelphia, PA 19104-4283, USA

L.H. Sobin
Head, WHO Collaborating Center
for the International Histological Classification of Tumours
Armed Forces Institute of Pathology
Washington, DC 20306-6000, USA

First edition published by WHO in 1974 as No. 12 in the International Histological Classification of Tumours series

ISBN-13: 978-3-540-60850-9

CIP data applied for

Die Deutsche Bibliothek — CIP-Einheitsaufnahme
International histological classification of tumours/World
Health Organization. — Berlin; Heidelberg; New York;
London; Paris; Tokyo; Hong Kong; Barcelona; Budapest:
Springer.
NE: World Health Organization
Heenan, Peter J.: Histological typing of skin tumours. — 2. ed. — 1996
Heenan, Peter J.:
Histological typing of skin tumours/authors: P.J. Heenan
and D.E. Elder. In collab. with L.H. Sobin and pathologists
in ten countries. [World Health Organization]. — 2. ed. — Berlin;
Heidelberg; New York; Barcelona; Budapest; Hong Kong;
London; Milan; Paris; Santa Clara; Singapore; Tokyo:
Springer, 1996
(International histological classification of tumours)
ISBN-13: 978-3-540-60850-9 e-ISBN-13: 978-3-642-80126-6
DOI: 10.1007/978-3-642-80126-6
NE: Elder, David E.:

Typesetting: Best-set Typesetter Ltd., Hong Kong

SPIN: 10523791 25/3130/SPS – 543210 – Printed on acid-free paper

Participants

Clark, W.H., Jr., Dr.
Beth Israel Hospital, Boston, USA

Elder, D.E., Dr.
Hospital of the University of Pennsylvania, Philadelphia, USA

Heenan, P.J., Dr.
The University of Western Australia, Perth, Australia

Hock Ong Beng, Dr.
Singapore General Hospital, Singapore

Kanitakis, J., Dr.
Hospital Edouard-Herriot, Lyon, France

Kirkham, N., Dr.
Royal Sussex County Hospital, Brighton, UK

Looi Lei Meng, Dr.
University of Malaya, Kuala Lumpur, Malaysia

Mishima, Y., Dr.
Kobe University School of Medicine, Kobe, Japan

Moreno, A., Dr.
Hospital Princeps d'Espanya, Barcelona, Spain

Murphy, G.F., Dr.
Hospital of the University of Pennsylvania, Philadelphia, USA

Rilke, F., Dr.
Istituto Nazionale Per Lo Studio E La Cura Dei Tumori,
Milan, Italy

Schmoeckel, C., Dr.
Munich, Germany

Sobin, L.H., Dr.
Armed Forces Institute of Pathology, Washington, DC, USA

Weedon, D., Dr.
Brisbane, Queensland, Australia

General Preface to the Series

Among the prerequisites for comparative studies of cancer are international agreement on histological criteria for the definition and classification of cancer types and a standardized nomenclature. An internationally agreed classification of tumours, acceptable alike to physicians, surgeons, radiologists, pathologists and statisticians, would enable cancer workers in all parts of the world to compare their findings and would facilitate collaboration among them.

In a report published in 1952,[1] a subcommittee of the World Health Organization (WHO) Expert Committee on Health Statistics discussed the general principles that should govern the statistical classification of tumours and agreed that, to ensure the necessary flexibility and ease of coding, three separate classifications were needed according to (1) anatomical site, (2) histological type and (3) degree of malignancy. A classification according to anatomical site is available in the International Classification of Diseases.[2]

In 1956, the WHO Executive Board passed a resolution[3] requesting the Director-General to explore the possibility that WHO might organize centres in various parts of the world and arrange for the collection of human tissues and their histological classification. The main purpose of such centres would be to develop histological definitions of cancer types and to facilitate the wide adoption of a uniform nomenclature. The resolution was endorsed by the Tenth World Health Assembly in May 1957.[4]

---

[1] WHO (1952) WHO Technical Report Series, No. 53, 1952, p. 45.

[2] WHO (1977) Manual of the international statistical classification of diseases, injuries, and causes of death, 1975 version, Geneva.

[3] WHO (1956) WHO Official Records. No. 68, p. 14 (resolution EB 17. R40).

[4] WHO (1957) WHO Official Records, No. 79, p. 467 (resolution WHA 10.18).

Since 1958, WHO has established a number of centres concerned with this subject. The result of this endeavour is the *International Histological Classification of Tumours*, a multivolume series whose first edition was published between 1967 and 1981. The present revised second edition aims to update the classification, reflecting progress in diagnosis and the relevance of tumour types to clinical and epidemiological features.

Preface to Histological Typing of Skin Tumours, Second Edition

The first edition of *Histological Typing of Skin Tumours*[1] was the result of a collaborative effort organized by WHO and carried out by the International Reference Centre for the Histological Classification of Skin Tumours at the Department of Pathology, University of Western Australia, Perth, Australia. The Reference Centre was established in 1965 and the Classification published in 1974.

In order to keep the Classification current, a new group of participants was appointed in 1990 which co-ordinated its activities from the Department of Pathology at the University of Western Australia. Drafts of the Classification were circulated to members of the group in ten countries for their comments, and the final version was produced by the co-authors and the series editor following discussions at the United States–Canadian Academy of Pathology Meeting in 1995. The histological classification of skin tumours contains the morphology code numbers of the International Classification of Diseases for Oncology (ICD-O)[2] and the Systematized Nomenclature of Medicine (SNOMED).[3] This classification, of course, reflects the present state of knowledge, and modifications will certainly be needed as experience accumulates and technological advances are incorporated into the daily practice of pathology. Although the present classification represents a consensus adopted by members of the group, it necessarily represents a view from which some patholo-

---

[1] ten Seldam REJ, Helwig EB, Sobin LH, Torloni H (1974) Histological typing of skin tumours. World Health Organization, Geneva (International Histological Classification of Tumours, No. 12).

[2] World Health Organization (1990) International Classification of Disease for Oncology. Geneva.

[3] College of American Pathologists (1982) Systematized Nomenclature of Medicine. Chicago.

gists may wish to dissent. It is our hope, nonetheless, that in the interests of international co-operation all pathologists will use the classification as put forward. Criticism and suggestions for its improvement will be welcomed; these should be sent to the World Health Organization, Geneva, Switzerland.

The publications in the series International Histological Classification of Tumours are not intended to serve as textbooks, but rather to promote the adoption of a uniform terminology that will facilitate communication among cancer workers. For this reason the literature references have intentionally been omitted and readers should refer to standard works for bibliographies.

Contents

Introduction

In the 21 years since the first edition of the *Histological Typing of Skin Tumours*, there have been major changes in skin tumour pathology, including the recognition of many new entities, changes in classifications and rapid advances in immunocytochemical diagnostic techniques. This edition has included the more important newly recognized skin tumours, resulting in considerable expansion in the categories of melanocytic and lymphoproliferative tumours, and including neoplasms of uncertain histogenesis such as primary cutaneous neuroendocrine carcinoma (Merkel cell tumour) and epithelioid sarcoma. The classification of melanoma in this edition is based on that of Clark, as presented in the Armed Forces Institute of Pathology *Atlas of Tumour Pathology*,[1] as discussed more fully in the introduction to the section on melanocytic tumours. Many soft tissue tumours defined and described in the second edition of *Histological Typing of Soft Tissue Tumours*[2] have not been further described in this volume, except for those tumours of major clinical importance that occur as primary tumours of cutaneous soft tissue.

As in the previous edition, the term "tumour" is used synonymously with "neoplasm". Some non-neoplastic lesions that may be confused both clinically and histologically with true neoplasms are therefore included. The classification is based primarily on differentiation as assessed by the light microscopic features of the tumours, rather than on histogenesis, although many of the definitions used have histogenetic implications.

---

[1] Elder DE, Murphy GF (1991) Melanocytic tumors of the skin. In: Atlas of tumor pathology. Armed Forces Institute of Pathology, Washington, D.C.

[2] Weiss SW (1994) Histological typing of soft tissue tumours, WHO International Histological Classification of Tumours. Springer-Verlag, Berlin Heidelberg New York.

Where important, reference is made in the explanatory notes to immunocytochemical reagents likely to be particularly helpful in differential diagnosis.

The text has been kept as brief as possible whilst attempting to incorporate accurate descriptions of the essential morphological features. The illustrations, mainly in black and white, are all new since the first edition.

Histological Classification of Skin Tumours

1 Melanocytic Tumours

1.1	*Benign (naevi)*	
1.1.1	Common acquired melanocytic naevi	
1.1.1.1	Lentigo simplex	57250[a]
1.1.1.2	Junctional melanocytic naevus	8740/0
1.1.1.3	Compound melanocytic naevus	8760/0
1.1.1.4	Dermal melanocytic naevus	8750/0
	Variants of acquired naevi	
1.1.1.5	Halo naevus	8723/0
1.1.1.6	Combined naevus	8720/0
1.1.1.7	Deep penetrating naevus	8720/0
1.1.1.8	Recurrent melanocytic naevus	8720/0
1.1.2	Spindle and epithelioid cell naevi	
1.1.2.1	Spitz naevus	8770/0
1.1.2.2	Pigmented spindle cell naevus of Reed	8770/0
1.1.3	Blue naevi	
1.1.3.1	Common blue naevus	8780/0
1.1.3.2	Cellular blue naevus	8790/0
1.1.4	Dermal melanocytoses	
1.1.4.1	Naevus of Ota	57240
1.1.4.2	Naevus of Ito	57230
1.1.4.3	Mongolian spot	57220
1.1.5	Congenital melanocytic naevi	
1.1.5.1	Small congenital naevi	8761/1
1.1.5.2	Intermediate and giant congenital naevi	8761/1
1.1.5.3	Proliferative dermal lesions in congenital naevi	8761/1

[a] Morphology code of the International Classificaton of Diseases for Oncology (ICD-O) and the Systematized Nomenclature of Medicine (SNOMED).

1.1.6	Dysplastic melanocytic naevi	
1.1.6.1	Junctional and compound dysplastic naevi	8727/0
1.2	*Malignant (melanomas and related lesions)*	
1.2.1	Superficial spreading melanoma	8743/3
1.2.2	Lentigo maligna	8742/2
1.2.3	Lentigo maligna melanoma	8742/3
1.2.4	Nodular melanoma	8721/3
1.2.5	Melanoma with unclassified epidermal component	8720/3
1.2.6	Acral-lentiginous melanoma	8744/3
1.2.7	Mucosal-lentiginous melanoma	8720/3
1.2.8	Desmoplastic melanoma	8745/3
1.2.9	Neurotropic melanoma	8745/3
1.2.10	Malignant blue naevus	8780/3
1.2.11	Melanoma in congenital melanocytic naevi	8761/3
1.2.12	Minimal deviation melanoma	8720/3
1.2.13	Clear cell sarcoma	9044/3
1.2.14	Malignant melanocytic schwannoma	9560/3
1.3	*Non-neoplastic hyperpigmentations*	
1.3.1	Ephelis (freckle)	57260
1.3.2	Solar (actinic) lentigo	57250
1.3.3	Mucosal melanosis (genital lentiginosis)	57210
1.3.4	Café au lait spot	57270

2 Epidermal Tumours

2.1	*Benign*	
2.1.1	Epidermal	
2.1.1.1	Epidermal naevus	75700
2.1.1.2	Seborrhoeic keratosis	72750
2.1.1.3	Clear cell acanthoma	72530
2.1.1.4	Fibroepithelial polyp (skin tag, acrochordon)	76810
2.1.1.5	Warty dyskeratoma (isolated dyskeratosis follicularis)	74450
2.1.1.6	Actinic keratosis (solar keratosis)	72850

2.1.1.7 Keratoacanthoma 72860
2.1.1.8 Benign lichenoid keratosis (lichen planus-like keratosis)
2.1.2 Verrucae (virus-related lesions)
2.1.2.1 Verruca vulgaris (common wart)........... 76630
2.1.2.2 Verruca plantaris (plantar wart)........... 76630
2.1.2.3 Verruca plana (flat wart) 76620
2.1.2.4 Condyloma acuminatum 76720
2.1.2.5 Giant condyloma acuminatum (Buschke and Lowenstein)................ 76730
2.1.2.6 Bowenoid papulosis
2.1.2.7 Molluscum contagiosum.................. 76660

2.2 *Malignant*
2.2.1 Squamous cell carcinoma................. 8070/3
Variants
2.2.1.1 Spindle cell squamous cell carcinoma 8074/3
2.2.1.2 Acantholytic squamous cell carcinoma 8070/3
2.2.1.3 Verrucous squamous cell carcinoma 8051/3
2.2.1.4 Squamous cell carcinoma with horn formation 8070/3
2.2.1.5 Lymphoepithelial squamous cell carcinoma 8082/3
2.2.2 Basal cell carcinoma 8090/3
Variants
2.2.2.1 Multifocal superficial basal cell carcinoma (superficial multicentric) 8091/3
2.2.2.2 Nodular basal cell carcinoma (solid, adenoid cystic) 8090/3
2.2.2.3 Infiltrating basal cell carcinoma 8090/3
2.2.2.3.1 Non-sclerosing 8090/3
2.2.2.3.2 Sclerosing (desmoplastic, morpheic) 8092/3
2.2.2.4 Fibroepithelial basal cell carcinoma 8093/3
2.2.2.5 Basal cell carcinoma with adnexal differentiation 8090/3
2.2.2.5.1 Follicular
2.2.2.5.2 Eccrine
2.2.2.6 Basosquamous carcinoma 8094/3
2.2.2.7 Keratotic basal cell carcinoma 8090/3
2.2.2.8 Pigmented basal cell carcinoma 8090/3

2.2.2.9	Basal cell carcinoma in basal cell naevus syndrome	8090/3
2.2.2.10	Micronodular basal cell carcinoma	8090/3

3 Adnexal Tumours

3.1	*Eccrine tumours*	
3.1.1	Benign	
3.1.1.1	Ciliated cyst	8400/0
3.1.1.2	Hidrocystoma (eccrine cystadenoma)	8404/0
3.1.1.3	Papillary eccrine adenoma	8408/0
3.1.1.4	Syringoma	8407/0
3.1.1.5	Mixed tumour of skin (chondroid syringoma)	8940/0
3.1.1.6	Eccrine poroma	8400/0
3.1.1.7	Syringofibroadenoma	8400/0
3.1.1.8	Nodular hidradenoma (eccrine acrospiroma, clear cell hidradenoma)	8402/0
3.1.1.9	Eccrine spiradenoma	8403/0
3.1.1.10	Cylindroma	8200/0
3.1.2	Malignant	
3.1.2.1	Sclerosing sweat duct carcinoma (syringomatous carcinoma, microcystic adnexal carcinoma)	8407/3
3.1.2.2	Malignant mixed tumour of the skin (malignant chondroid syringoma)	8940/3
3.1.2.3	Porocarcinoma	8400/3
3.1.2.4	Malignant nodular hidradenoma	8402/3
3.1.2.5	Malignant eccrine spiradenoma	8403/3
3.1.2.6	Mucinous eccrine carcinoma	8480/3
3.1.2.7	Adenoid cystic eccrine carcinoma	8200/3
3.1.2.8	Aggressive digital papillary adenoma/adenocarcinoma	

3.2	*Apocrine tumours*	
3.2.1	Benign	
3.2.1.1	Apocrine cystadenoma (hidrocystoma)	8401/0
3.2.1.2	Hidradenoma papilliferum	8405/0
3.2.1.3	Syringocystadenoma papilliferum	8406/0
3.2.1.4	Apocrine adenoma	8401/0

3.2.1.5	Cylindroma	8200/0
3.2.2	Malignant	
3.2.2.1	Apocrine adenocarcinoma	8401/3
3.3	*Sebaceous gland tumours*	
3.3.1	Benign	
3.3.1.1	Sebaceous adenoma	8410/0
3.3.1.2	Sebaceous epithelioma	
3.3.2	Malignant	
3.3.2.1	Sebaceous carcinoma	8410/3
3.3.3	Pilosebaceous hyperplasia and hamartomas	
3.3.3.1	Follicular naevi	75500
3.3.3.2	Naevus sebaceus	75750
3.3.3.3	Sebaceous gland hyperplasia	72000
3.4	*Hair follicle tumours*	
3.4.1	Benign	
3.4.1.1	Conical infundibular acanthoma (dilated pore)	
3.4.1.2	Pilar sheath acanthoma	
3.4.1.3	Trichilemmoma	8102/0
3.4.1.4	Tumour of follicular infundibulum	
3.4.1.5	Trichoepithelioma	8100/0
3.4.1.6	Trichofolliculoma	8101/0
3.4.1.7	Pilomatricoma	8110/0
3.4.1.8	Pilar tumour (proliferating trichilemmal cyst)	72670
3.4.2	Malignant	
3.4.2.1	Trichilemmocarcinoma	8102/3
3.4.2.2	Malignant pilomatricoma (matrical carcinoma)	8110/3
3.4.3	Follicular cysts	
3.4.3.1	Infundibular cyst	33430
3.4.3.2	Trichilemmal cyst (pilar cyst)	33470
3.4.3.3	Steatocystoma multiplex	33450
3.4.3.4	Dermoid cyst	9084/0
3.4.3.5	Eruptive vellus hair cyst	33400
3.4.4	Tumours of pilosebaceous mesenchyme	
3.4.4.1	Follicular fibroma (trichodiscoma, fibrofolliculoma, perifollicular fibroma)	

4 Paget Disease

4.1	*Mammary Paget disease*	8541/3
4.2	*Extramammary Paget disease*	8542/3

5 Cutaneous Lymphoproliferative Tumours

5.1	*Cutaneous T-cell lymphoma*	
5.1.1	Mycosis fungoides	9700/3
5.1.2	Sezary syndrome	9701/3
5.1.3	Pagetoid reticulosis (Woringer-Kollop disease)	9700/3
5.1.4	Adult T-cell lymphoma/leukaemia	9827/3
5.2	*Cutaneous B-cell lymphoma*	9709/3
5.3	*Cutaneous plasmacytoma*	9731/3
5.4	*Cutaneous lymphoma, pleomorphic variants*	
5.4.1	T-immunoblastic lymphoma	9684/3
5.4.2	Large cell anaplastic lymphoma	9714/3
5.5	*Dysplastic lymphocytic proliferations* (lymphomatoid vasculitis)	
5.5.1	Lymphomatoid papulosis	72230
5.5.2	Lymphomatoid granulomatosis	9766/1
5.5.3	Angioimmunoblastic lymphadenopathy	9767/1
5.6	*Langerhans cell histiocytosis (histiocytosis X)*	77910
5.7	*Regressing atypical histiocytosis*	77800
5.8	*Mastocytosis*	9740/1
5.9	*Leukaemia cutis*	9800/3

6 Vascular Tumours

6.1	*Benign*	
6.1.1	Capillary haemangioma	9131/0
6.1.2	Cavernous haemangioma	9121/0
6.1.3	Angiokeratoma	9141/0
6.1.4	Verrucous keratotic haemangioma	9142/0
6.1.5	Tufted haemangioma	9120/0
6.1.6	Spindle cell angioendothelioma	9130/1

6.1.7	Glomus tumour	8711/0
6.1.8	Glomangioma	8712/0
6.2	*Malignant*	
6.2.1	Kaposi sarcoma	9140/3
6.2.2	Angiosarcoma	9120/3
6.3	*Vascular malformations*	24600
6.3.1	Naevus flammeus	75540
6.3.2	Hereditary haemorrhagic telangiectasia	
6.3.3	Angioma serpiginosum	
6.4	*Vascular hyperplasias*	72570
6.4.1	Acroangiodermatitis	
6.4.2	Intravascular papillary endothelial hyperplasia	
6.4.3	Bacillary angiomatosis	76316
6.4.4	Pyogenic granuloma (lobular haemangioma, haemangioma of granulation tissue type)	44440
6.4.5	Angiolymphoid hyperplasia with eosinophilia (epithelioid haemangioma)	72260

7 Lymphatic Tumours

7.1	*Benign*	
7.1.1	Capillary lymphangioma	9171/0
7.1.2	Cavernous lymphangioma	9172/0
7.1.3	Cystic lymphangioma (hygroma)	9173/0
7.2	*Malignant*	
7.2.1	Lymphangiosarcoma (malignant lymphangioendothelioma)	9170/3

8 Cutaneous Fibrohistiocytic Tumours

8.1	*Benign*	
8.1.1	Benign fibrous histiocytoma (dermatofibroma, histiocytoma, sclerosing haemangioma)	8830/0
	Variants	

8.1.1.1	Cellular benign fibrous histiocytoma	
8.1.1.2	Aneurysmal benign fibrous histiocytoma	
8.1.1.3	Epithelioid benign fibrous histiocytoma	
8.1.1.4	Atypical (pseudosarcomatous) benign fibrous histiocytoma	
8.1.2	Dermatomyofibroma	
8.1.3	Benign (juvenile) xanthogranuloma	55380
8.1.4	Reticulohistiocytoma	77880
8.1.5	Xanthoma	55300
8.2	*Malignant*	
8.2.1	Atypical fibroxanthoma	8830/1
8.2.2	Dermatofibrosarcoma protuberans	8832/3
8.2.3	Malignant fibrous histiocytoma	8830/3
8.3	*Angiofibromatous proliferations*	
8.3.1	Adenoma sebaceum	75730
8.3.2	Fibrous papule	9160/0
8.4	*Digital mesenchymal tumours*	
8.4.1	Digital fibroma	76100
8.4.2	Digital fibrokeratoma	8810/0
8.4.3	Digital mucous cyst	8840/0
8.5	*Dermal mesenchymal tumours of infancy and childhood*	
8.5.1	Infantile myofibromatosis	8824/1
8.5.2	Fibrous hamartoma of infancy	75560
8.5.3	Naevus lipomatosus superficialis	75760
8.5.4	Juvenile hyaline fibromatosis	
8.5.5	Giant cell fibroblastoma	
8.6	*Plexiform fibrohistiocytic tumour*	

9 Nervous Tissue Tumours

9.1	*Benign*	
9.1.1	Neurofibroma	9540/0
9.1.2	Neurilemoma	9560/0
9.1.3	Granular cell tumour	9580/0

9.1.4	Dermal nerve sheath myxoma and neurothekeoma	9562/0
9.1.5	Palisaded encapsulated neuroma (solitary neuroma)	9570/0
9.1.6	Pacinian neurofibroma (pacinioma)	9507/0
9.2	*Malignant*	
9.2.1	Malignant schwannoma	9560/3
9.2.2	Malignant granular cell tumour	9580/3

10 Tumours of Muscle

10.1	*Benign*	
10.1.1	Piloleiomyoma	8890/0
10.1.2	Angioleiomyoma	8894/0
10.2	*Malignant*	
10.2.1	Superficial leiomyosarcoma	8890/3

11 Miscellaneous Tumours

11.1	*Primary cutaneous neuroendocrine carcinoma (Merkel cell tumour)*	8247/3
11.2	*Epithelioid sarcoma*	8804/3

Definitions and Explanatory Notes

1 Melanocytic Tumours

Introduction

Malignant Melanoma

In the First Edition of the World Health Organization (WHO) *Histological Typing of Skin Tumours* (1974), malignant melanoma was classified into four categories:

1. Malignant melanoma
2. Malignant melanoma arising in precancerous melanosis, including Hutchinson's melanotic freckle
3. Malignant melanoma arising in a blue naevus
4. Malignant melanoma arising in giant pigmented naevus

Most melanomas, according to this classification, would belong to categories 1 and 2, the essential histological difference between the two types being the presence of "precancerous melanosis including Hutchinson's melanotic freckle" in the epidermis adjacent to the invasive neoplasm in category 2, whereas in category 1 there was no such adjacent component.

In the ensuing years, however, the clinicopathological classification of Clark has become widely accepted. The classification used in this second edition of the *Histological Typing of Skin Tumours* is based on the original classification of Clark and is essentially the same as that proposed in the current Armed Forces Institute of Pathology (AFIP) fascicle on skin tumours. In this classification, nodular melanoma is equivalent to the previous category 1, "malignant melanoma". The previous category 2, "malignant melanoma arising in precancerous melanosis including Hutchinson's melanotic freckle", is separated into malignant melanoma of superficial spreading or pagetoid type and lentigo malignant melanoma, or malignant melanoma developing in

Hutchinson's melanotic freckle. Additional categories not included in the first edition are desmoplastic and neurotropic melanoma, acral-lentiginous melanoma, mucosal-lentiginous melanoma and melanoma of unclassified histological type.

It is acknowledged that some authorities believe that there is probably no essential biological difference between some or perhaps all of these categories of melanoma. In particular, it is likely that nodular melanoma is a variant of the commonest form of melanoma, i.e. superficial spreading melanoma, in which expansile growth of the neoplastic cells has produced the characteristic nodule which has overgrown the pre-existing adjacent component. Nodules also occur in other categories, including lentigo maligna melanoma, indicating a similar risk of metastasis regardless of the histological type of melanoma. The widespread acceptance of this classification, however, has been based on its clinicopathological correlations, on the results of epidemiological studies that have indicated possible aetiological differences between some subtypes and on the didactic value of recognizing morphologic variations as an aid to the diagnostic process.

The recognition that melanomas with invasion of the papillary dermis by smaller groups of melanocytes than those present within the epidermis apparently do not have the potential to metastasize has led to the introduction of the term *radial growth phase* for these non-metastasizing melanomas with microscopic dermal invasion. Synonyms for this phase in melanoma development are *plaque phase* and *non-tumorigenic melanoma.* For those melanomas that have acquired the capacity to proliferate in the dermis and form a mass, the terms *vertical growth phase* and *tumorigenic* have been introduced. These tumours include those in which there is invasion of the papillary dermis by neoplastic melanocytes arranged in groups larger than those in the epidermis. Tumorigenic melanoma may have competence for metastasis, but this is vanishingly rare in the non-tumorigenic radial growth phase. Further discussion of these concepts of the biological potential of melanoma is beyond the scope of this volume, in which attention is concentrated on the diagnostic morphological features of melanoma.

In Situ Melanoma

The term in situ melanoma may be applied to the patterns of intra-epidermal melanocytic proliferation seen in lentigo maligna (Hutchinson's melanotic freckle), superficial spreading (pagetoid melanoma), acral-lentiginous and mucosal-lentiginous melanoma. The histological criteria for in situ melanoma recommended in this classification are as follows:

1. Atypical melanocytes in a confluent linear pattern along the dermo-epidermal junction with or without nest formation (lentiginous pattern).
2. Infiltration of part or the full thickness of the epidermis by atypical epithelioid melanocytes arranged singly or in groups (superficial spreading, pagetoid pattern). In tumours with less florid proliferation of less atypical melanocytes, disposed in an intermittent pattern along the basal layer, extending in some cases as scattered single cells in the lower layers of the stratum malpighii without classical pagetoid infiltration and without uniform cytologic atypia, alternative terms such as intra-epidermal or intra-epithelial melanocytic atypia might reasonably be used.

Precursor Melanocytic Lesions

The concept of intra-epithelial cellular atypia followed by progression, in an unknown proportion of cases, to in situ and ultimately, again in an unknown proportion of cases, to invasion is generally accepted as being of fundamental importance in the pathogenesis of neoplasia in epithelia such as those of the cervix and of the colon in the adenoma–carcinoma sequence. When applied to melanocytic neoplasia, this general concept of tumour progression suggests the acceptance of the existence of precursor or premalignant melanocytic lesions, including the *dysplastic naevus* and other atypical intra-epidermal melanocytic proliferations. The dysplastic naevus concept, although controversial, has been widely accepted as a means of identifying, by clinical and histological criteria, those melanocytic lesions whose biological potential appears to lie between that of common acquired naevi and malignant melanoma. While it is acknowledged that the term dysplasia in this context is not universally approved, its use in this volume is in accordance with the second editions of the WHO Histological Typing of Tumours in other systems in this series, where dysplasia is employed as a term that can be used to describe most precancerous epithelial lesions. A precancerous lesion is described by the authors of the volume on the *Histological Typing of Oesophageal and Gastric Tumours* as a histopathological abnormality that is more likely to develop into cancer than its normal counterpart, while not implying that malignant progression in such a lesion is inevitable; rather it is a marker of an increased probability of malignant change. Dysplastic naevus is included in this classification, therefore, as a marker for increased risk of developing melanoma and as a possible precursor of malignant melanoma.

1.1 Benign (naevi)

1.1.1 Common acquired melanocytic naevi

Acquired melanocytic naevi are benign neoplasms of epidermal melanocytes. These lesions first appear in early childhood, reaching a maximum size in adolescence and tending to disappear in later life. Melanocytic naevi comprise a range of neoplasms distinguished by different patterns of growth of altered melanocytes which are considerably larger than normal melanocytes. These cells have much more abundant cytoplasm than their normal counterparts and tend to retain melanin. They are non-dendritic and usually of rounded or epithelioid shape. The earliest recognizable lesion is the simple lentigo, clinically a small (usually less than 4 mm in diameter), flat or very slightly raised, darkly pigmented lesion with sharply defined borders. The term is derived from the resemblance of the small lesions to a lentil (seed). Histologically, these lesions are characterized by a linear pattern of contiguous altered melanocytes along the basal layer of the epidermis, usually with elongation of the rete ridges and without nest formation. This pattern, which is recapitulated in some melanomas, is termed "lentiginous". The next step in the uninterrupted life history of melanocytic naevi is the development of nests of these melanocytes at the dermo-epidermal junction, forming the junctional naevus, which is also usually flat or only slightly raised. In the next stage of development, nests of melanocytes migrate from the dermo-epidermal junction into the papillary dermis, forming a compound naevus. As more nests of junctional melanocytes migrate into the papillary dermis, the older melanocytes descend further into the dermis, where they become smaller and usually more diffusely arranged. The speed with which this process occurs varies, but usually the lifespan of a common acquired naevus is one of many years. Eventually all of the altered intra-epidermal melanocytes (naevus cells) migrate into the dermis, and the lesion is then known as an intradermal or dermal naevus. Over a further period, usually of many years, intradermal naevi involute so that in old age many acquired naevi disappear.

1.1.1.1 Lentigo simplex (Fig. 1)

A localized area of linear proliferation of melanocytes along the dermo-epidermal junction without nest formation.

The epidermis shows elongation of the rete ridges with hyperpigmentation of the basal layer and enlarged, non-dendritic melanocytes in a linear pattern along the basal layer of the epidermis, forming confluent rows. Lentigo is distinguished from a freckle by the presence of melanocytic proliferation as well as hyperpigmentation, and from a junctional naevus by the absence of nest formation.

Simple lentigines are small (up to 5 mm), flat pigmented lesions with sharply defined borders. They occur on all cutaneous surfaces, but tend to be concentrated more on exposed areas. The natural history of lentigines is to remain stable for long periods or to develop into junctional naevi. Regression also occurs.

1.1.1.2 Junctional melanocytic naevus (Fig. 2)

A benign neoplasm of epidermal melanocytes arranged as single cells and in nests along the dermo-epidermal junction.

In addition to the features of simple lentigo, there are nests of melanocytes at the dermo-epidermal junction, mainly at the bases of elongated rete ridges.

Junctional naevi are small (usually less than 5 mm in diameter), flat or slightly raised, symmetrical lesions found on any cutaneous surface.

1.1.1.3 Compound melanocytic naevus (Fig. 3)

A melanocytic naevus in which, in addition to naevus cells at the dermo-epidermal junction, naevus cells are also present in the dermis.

Nests of variably pigmented melanocytes, usually epithelioid, are present at the dermo-epidermal junction and in the dermis to varying depths. The epithelium is often hyperplastic with elongation of the rete ridges and hyperpigmentation of the basal layer. In the dermis, the melanocytes are arranged in nests and strands, separated by a delicate stroma and becoming smaller and more diffusely arranged in the deeper layers. This pattern of "maturation" may be expressed as the transition from the superficial type A epithelioid naevus cell to the deeper type B smaller, non-pigmented cell. A third type of cell, the type C spindle cell, is sometimes present at the base of older lesions.

Compound naevi are usually small (less than 10 mm in diameter), and their profile may be flat, papular or papillomatous. The lesion is usually circumscribed and asymmetrical with a regular border and uniformly tan or brown, less commonly pink or flesh-coloured pigmentation.

1.1.1.4 Dermal melanocytic naevus (Figs. 4, 5)

A melanocytic naevus in which the naevus cells are virtually confined to the dermis. A few naevus cells are frequently found, however, at the dermo-epidermal junction.

Nests of epithelioid and multinucleated giant melanocytes are present in the papillary dermis, often extending into the reticular dermis, becoming smaller and more attenuated in the deeper layers, where the cells are arranged singly and in slender strands. Neurotization is frequently present where structures resembling Meissner corpuscles are formed, and the deep spindle cells may be arranged in parallel bundles in a fibrillar stroma, resembling neurofibroma.

These naevi are circumscribed, variably pigmented papules tending to become flatter and eventually to disappear over a period of decades in a process of involution.

Balloon cell change (Fig. 6). In some naevi, variable proportions of naevus cells have greatly expanded clear cytoplasm due to the presence of multiple vacuoles, probably abnormal melanosomes. This feature may be seen in otherwise unremarkable naevi and in melanomas; it has no known clinical significance. If the lesion is composed mainly of balloon cells, the term *balloon cell naevus* can be used.

Naevus of genital skin. *A benign melanocytic naevus of junctional, compound or intradermal type occurring on the genital skin.*

These are usually small, asymmetrical, circumscribed naevi in which there is some variation in the size and shape of junctional nests of cells, which may be arranged parallel to the surface of the epidermis. The naevus cells may have large, pleomorphic nuclei with prominent nucleoli. These features can cause confusion with melanoma, but there is little or no infiltration of the epidermis by atypical melanocytes, the junctional component does not extend laterally beyond the dermal component, mitoses are absent and the deeper dermal naevus cells are smaller, indicating maturation.

1.1.1.5 Halo naevus (Sutton naevus, leukoderma acquisitum) (Fig. 7)

A melanocytic naevus surrounded by a symmetrical zone of depigmentation.

A lymphocytic infiltrate, often very dense, is present in the stroma of the naevus, with disappearance of naevus cells progressively as the lymphocytic infiltrate becomes denser and more extensive, ultimately leaving a fibrotic scar and scattered melanophages in the dermis at the site of complete regression of the naevus. The epidermis in the halo region shows reduction in pigmentation with a sparse superficial lymphohistiocytic infiltrate in the dermis. Residual naevus cells in these lesions may be larger than usual in common naevi, with prominent nucleoli, representing inflammatory or reactive atypia.

1.1.1.6 Combined naevus (Fig. 8)

A melanocytic naevus in which the usual epithelioid naevus cells are combined with a component of pigmented spindle cells arranged singly and in strands between collagen bundles, as in blue naevi. Spitz naevus (spindle and epithelioid cell naevus) may also be combined with a common naevus.

1.1.1.7 Deep penetrating naevus (Fig. 9)

A benign acquired melanocytic naevus with mixed features of blue naevus, combined naevus and Spitz naevus.

The tumours are composed of large, variably pigmented, spindle and epithelioid melanocytes forming sparse junctional nests, extending into the deep reticular dermis and often into subcutaneous fat, arranged in small nests and fascicles with melanophages in the adjacent stroma. Groups of smaller epithelioid naevus cells are also present in some tumours. At the periphery of the lesion, the nests of cells are more dispersed. The nuclei are frequently pleomorphic and vacuolated and may contain large eosinophilic nucleoli. The cells at the base of the tumour may be as large as those in the superficial layers, but mitoses are absent or rare and there is little associated stromal reaction.

These recently described naevi occur most commonly on the head, neck and shoulder from early childhood to late adult life. The deeply pigmented papular or nodular lesions are usually diagnosed clinically as blue naevus or cellular blue naevus. They may be misdiagnosed histologically as malignant melanoma.

1.1.1.8 Recurrent melanocytic naevus (Fig. 10)

Recurrent melanocytic naevus (pseudomelanoma) represents persistence of a melanocytic lesion as the result of incomplete removal of a naevus, usually following attempted shave excision.

Junctional melanocytic nests of varied size and shape, tending to confluence, and the presence of melanocytes singly and in nests above the dermo-epidermal junction are features similar to those of in situ melanoma. The features indicating the benign nature of the lesions, however, are the absence of severe cytological atypia, predominance of nests of cells over single cells in the epidermis, and absent or rare mitoses. Fibrosis is usually present in the superficial dermis, and the melanocytes deep to the scar are of bland morphology. The atypical melanocytes in the epidermis seldom extend beyond the lateral border of the scar, an important feature distinguishing them from recurrent melanoma.

Recurrent naevi usually follow incomplete removal of intradermal or compound melanocytic naevi. Paradoxically, recurrence of a naevus occurs over a few weeks, while recurrence of a melanoma is much slower (months to years).

1.1.2 Spindle and epithelioid cell naevi

1.1.2.1 Spitz naevus (Figs. 11, 12)

Benign melanocytic naevi of junctional, compound or intradermal distribution, composed of large spindle and/or epithelioid melanocytes.

Spitz naevi are symmetrical, sharply circumscribed melanocytic neoplasms, usually less than 6mm in diameter, although larger variants more than 10mm in diameter do occur. The epidermis is usually markedly hyperplastic, overlying junctional nests of epithelioid and/or spindle cells, often separated from the adjacent keratinocytes by peripheral clefts. The junctional nests of melanocytes are sometimes oriented vertically. Scattered single melanocytes may be present in the upper layers of the epidermis. In compound Spitz naevi, similar nests and fascicles of melanocytes are present in the superficial dermis, but in the deeper dermis the cells are usually distributed in a more diffuse pattern, singly and in small groups between the collagen bundles. The cells at the base of the tumour are usually smaller than those in the upper layers, suggesting maturation. They extend among reticular dermal collagen bundles as dispersed single cells, with "outlier cells" extending far from the main tumour mass. Melanomas, in contrast, tend to invade as more cohesive fascicles. The cells of Spitz naevi can sometimes be seen in the walls of appendages, including arrector pili muscles, without destroying them. A perivascular lymphocytic infiltrate is frequently present in the stroma, and the papillary dermis usually contains dilated blood vessels. Eosinophilic globules (Kamino bodies) are frequently present in the epidermis and at the dermo-epidermal junction overlying Spitz naevi.

In tumours composed mainly of epithelioid cells, multinucleated giant cells are frequently present in the superficial layers, but their nuclei are usually relatively uniform. Mitoses may be seen, although only in small numbers and usually confined to the upper third of the neoplasm. The presence of multiple nests of large epithelioid melanocytes in these lesions at the dermo-epidermal junction and along the sides of elongated, interlocking rete ridges in zones of complex epidermal hyperplasia may result in apparent invasion of the epidermis by some of these nests, which, combined with scattered single tumour cells above the basal layer, may present an appearance suggestive of genuine pagetoid invasion of the epidermis, as seen in malignant melanoma of the superficial spreading type. In the absence of other diagnostic features of melanoma, however, this pattern of growth, when seen immediately above a tumour with other typical features of Spitz naevus, does not signify malignancy. The large epithelioid cells of Spitz naevus have abundant pale eosinophilic or amphophilic cytoplasm and large nuclei, often with prominent eosinophilic nucleoli and nuclear pseudovacuoles.

Some Spitz naevi are larger, polypoid tumours greater than 10mm in diameter and may be composed of large epithelioid cells showing little or no maturation in the deeper layers. Symmetry and sharp circumscription of the tumour, uniformity of nuclei (although they may be large with prominent nucleoli) and sparsity of mitoses in these larger tumours are helpful features to distinguish them from malignant melanoma. Some Spitz naevi are entirely intradermal in their distribution (dermal Spitz naevus).

Desmoplastic Spitz naevus. This variant of Spitz naevus is composed of spindle and epithelioid cells arranged in small groups and singly in the dermis separated by desmoplastic stroma. The lesions are symmetrical, and the tumour cells mature with descent into the dermis.

Although diagnosed most frequently in childhood, Spitz naevi may occur at any age. A common presentation is that of a rapidly growing pink papule on the face of a child, clinically resembling pyogenic granuloma or haemangioma. Spitz naevi are usually solitary, but multiple lesions may also develop on normal skin or in a macule similar to a "café au lait" spot. This variant is known as the agminate form of Spitz naevus.

1.1.2.2 Pigmented spindle cell naevus of Reed (Fig. 13)

A small, circumscribed tumour of heavily pigmented spindle-shaped melanocytes at the dermo-epidermal junction and, sometimes, in the papillary dermis.

The epidermis is hyperplastic, with pigmentation of keratinocytes; a patchy lymphocytic infiltrate and scattered melanophages may be present in the papillary dermis. These tumours sometimes include a smaller proportion of plump epithelioid cells, similar to those of Spitz naevi, which tend to become smaller when they are present in the papillary dermis. Mitoses may be seen in the junctional melanocytes, but they are rare in the dermis, where their presence suggests the possibility of melanoma. This tumour shares features in common with Spitz naevus and is also known as pigmented Spitz naevus.

Pigmented spindle cell naevi occur in both sexes, often on the lower limbs of young women, but also on all cutaneous surfaces.

1.1.3 Blue naevi

1.1.3.1 Common blue naevus (Fig. 14)

A tumour composed of heavily pigmented spindle-shaped and dendritic melanocytes located mainly in the reticular dermis.

The spindle and dendritic cells are distributed singly and in strands between the collagen bundles of the dermis, frequently arranged parallel to the epidermal surface in the superficial layers. The degree of pigmentation varies, but most tumours contain many cells with abundant coarse melanin granules. The degree of cellularity also varies, including some tumours in which the cells are widely dispersed. Some tumours extend into the subcutis.

Blue naevi are sharply circumscribed, flat or nodular lesions usually 4–15 mm in diameter and of bluish-black colour. They occur most commonly on the face and upper limb, but may occur anywhere on the skin.

1.1.3.2 Cellular blue naevus (Fig. 15)

A relatively large tumour composed of densely packed, variably pigmented spindle cells in the dermis.

These tumours are composed of densely packed nodules of dendritic and plumper spindle cells, often extending through the full thickness of the dermis into the subcutis, presenting a dumb-bell shape. A biphasic pattern of lightly pigmented or clear cells alternating with heavily pigmented spindle cells is a characteristic feature. An alveolar pattern may be presented by groups of clear spindle cells surrounded by heavily pigmented tumour cells. In the neuronaevoid growth pattern, the spindle cells are arranged in intertwining fascicles resembling peripheral nerves. In some tumours nuclear pleomorphism may be pronounced with large nucleoli, but mitoses are rare and necrosis is not seen. The rarity of mitoses, the absence of necrosis and the presence of dendritic cells are points in favour of a benign nature.

Cellular blue naevi are bluish-black, circumscribed, nodular tumours most often found in the lower lumbo-sacral region and the acral extremities. The cut surface is usually brownish black, very firm and sometimes gritty in consistency. Regional lymph node metastasis from apparently benign cellular blue naevi involving only the peripheral sinus of the lymph node is a rare, but well documented phenomenon which has been associated with a favourable prognosis. Lymph node metastasis with replacement of parenchyma by atypical cells, however, indicates that the primary tumour should best be regarded as a malignant blue naevus.

1.1.4 Dermal melanocytoses (naevus of Ota, naevus of Ito, Mongolian spot) (Fig. 16)

Macular, purplish blue–brown lesions composed of dendritic and/or spindle-shaped pigmented melanocytes between the collagen bundles of the reticular dermis.

Heavily pigmented dendritic melanocytes are distributed diffusely and often inconspicuously in the reticular dermis, arranged parallel to the epidermis between the collagen bundles around appendages. There is no epidermal melanocytic proliferation, but the epidermis may be hyperpigmented. The *naevus of Ota* is indistinguishable histologically from the *naevus of Ito* (dermal melanocytosis of the shoulder region). In the *Mongolian spot*, the melanocytes tend to be larger, more numerous and located in the deeper dermis, whereas the cells of the naevi of Ota and of Ito are present in the superficial reticular dermis.

The Mongolian spot and the naevi of Ota and Ito are classified clinically according to their anatomical distribution. The naevus of Ota is a congenital or acquired hyperpigmentation of the skin of the face and ocular mucous membranes in the distribution of branches of the trigeminal nerve, also known as ocular dermal melanocytosis. The naevus of Ito occurs on the shoulder region, whereas the Mongolian spot is found in sacrococcygeal skin. In the naevus of Ota, malignancy occasionally develops in the meninges, orbit and occasionally in the skin, forming dermal and subcutaneous masses.

1.1.5 Congenital melanocytic naevi

Melanocytic naevi that are present at birth. These are subdivided by size as follows: small congenital naevi, i.e. those up to 1.5 cm in diameter; giant congenital naevi, which typically cover large areas of the body (garment naevi, bathing trunk naevi) and are not as a rule amenable to complete surgical excision; and intermediate congenital naevi, i.e. those between the other groups.

1.1.5.1 Small congenital naevi (Fig. 17)

Nests of melanocytes are present at the dermo-epidermal junction and/or in the dermis, often extending into the deep dermis, arranged around and sometimes within the walls of appendages and around blood vessels. Small naevus cells are sometimes arranged between the collagen bundles in a very diffuse, splayed pattern. These features are not seen in all congenital naevi, many of which may be indistinguishable from common acquired naevi.

1.1.5.2 Intermediate and giant congenital naevi

The appearances in the superficial dermis are similar to those of common acquired naevi and small congenital naevi. The naevus cells in giant naevi, however, characteristically extend into the deep reticular dermis and often into the subcutis in a diffuse pattern where individual naevus cells are splayed between the collagen bundles. The deep naevus cells are usually small, resembling fibroblasts. Giant naevi frequently include areas with neuroid differentiation composed of fascicles of wavy fibres and naevus cells suggestive of neural structures, neurofibroma-like areas, cartilage and pseudo-Meissner corpuscles. Foci resembling blue naevi and cellular blue naevi also occur.

1.1.5.3 Proliferative dermal lesions in congenital naevi (Fig. 18)

Nodular areas may be present at birth or develop during later life in congenital naevi, most commonly in the giant type. These nodules are usually small, less than 5 mm in diameter and may be multiple; they usually comprise areas of denser cellularity than in the remainder of the naevus, often including larger, heavily pigmented spindle shaped cells, similar to cellular blue naevi. In most cases these nodular areas appear to blend with the surrounding naevus and are benign.

1.1.6 Dysplastic melanocytic naevi

1.1.6.1 Junctional and compound dysplastic naevi (atypical naevus, naevus with architectural disorder and melanocytic atypia) (Fig. 19)

A variant of an acquired naevus that is clinically atypical and characterized histologically by the combination of an immature (lentiginous) architectural pattern of melanocytic proliferation in the epidermis and cytologic atypia.

Dysplastic melanocytic naevi may be either junctional or compound. The junctional dysplastic naevus is a flat or slightly elevated lentiginous lesion with no associated papular compound naevus. The compound dysplastic naevus combines a central benign compound naevus with a peripheral lentiginous component. The typical changes of melanocytic dysplasia are found in the lentiginous junctional component, although dysplasia may also extend into the epidermis above a dermal component. The dysplasia usually extends for several rete ridges beyond the dermal naevus cells. The majority of melanocytes in dysplastic naevi are similar to those of banal naevi, i.e. naevoid melanocytes, larger than normal melanocytes, mainly round with sparse cytoplasm, with cytoplasmic retraction in some cells, and scanty coarse melanin pigment. The more atypical cytological features are present in a minority of tumour cells which are larger than most common naevus cells, with more abundant cytoplasm, i.e. epithelioid cells. The nuclei are more pleomorphic, some being small and pyknotic, whereas others are larger with irregular nuclear membranes, and some have prominent nucleoli. Finely granular, dusty melanin pigment may be seen in the cytoplasm of some cells. Cytological atypia may be slight or severe, depending on the degrees of nuclear pleomorphism, nuclear size, hyperchromasia and abnormal nucleoli. Mitoses are rare and there is little, if any, pagetoid infiltration of the epidermis. These more atypical epithelioid melanocytes form a minority of the cell population, arranged in intermittent distribution as single cells or small nests between the banal naevus cells (random cytologic atypia). Confluent growth of these more atypical epithelioid cells with pagetoid invasion of the epidermis, on the other hand, is diagnostic of in situ melanoma. The rete ridges in these lentiginous areas are elongated and the nests of melanocytes are varied in size and shape, often oriented with their long axis parallel to the epidermal surface, with bridging between adjacent rete ridges in some areas. In melanomas, the rete ridge pattern is often effaced with irregular thickening and thinning of the epidermis. Dermal stromal changes that accompany the cytological atypia of dysplastic naevi are characteristic, but not specific. A sparse lymphocytic infiltrate is present in the papillary dermis with condensed collagen (eosinophilic fibroplasia) around the bases of the elongated rete ridges. Another, less common, pattern of fibroplasia (lamellar fibroplasia) shows plates of collagen and spindle cells immediately below the bases of elongated rete ridges.

According to a 1985 conference sponsored by the World Health Organization,[1] major histological criteria for the diagnosis of dysplastic naevus are as follows:

---

[1] Clemente C, Cochran A, Elder DE et al (1991) Histopathologic diagnosis of dysplastic nevi. Concordance among pathologists convened by the WHO melanoma programme. Hum Pathol 22: 313–319.

1. Basilar proliferation of atypical melanocytes extending at least three rete ridges beyond the dermal naevocellular naevus
2. Lentiginous or epithelioid cell pattern of the atypical intra-epidermal melanocytic proliferation

Minor criteria include two or more of the following: concentric eosinophilic fibrosis or lamellar fibroplasia, neovascularization, dermal inflammatory host response, fusion of rete ridges.

Dysplastic naevi are larger (usually more than 5 mm) and more irregular in outline than common acquired naevi. The degree of pigmentation may be varied, but they are often mottled brown lesions with ill-defined borders. In profile, the lesions are either flat or present a combination of a flat macular component surrounding a central elevated papule.

1.2 Malignant (melanomas and related lesions)

1.2.1 **Superficial spreading melanoma** (Figs. 20, 21)

A neoplasm of atypical epithelioid melanocytes arranged in pagetoid pattern within the epidermis and invading the dermis.

The diagnosis of superficial spreading melanoma is made only when the pagetoid intra-epidermal component extends laterally beyond the invasive and tumorigenic component; otherwise, the lesion is a nodular melanoma. The cells are large, with varied cytoplasmic pigmentation, characteristically arranged in fine, dusty granules. In the plaque or radial growth phase, the groups of melanoma cells in the dermis are smaller than those in the epidermis, and mitoses are absent. In tumorigenic or vertical growth phase, which may occur even when the invasive tumour is confined to the papillary dermis without filling or expanding it (level 2), a group or groups of tumour cells in the dermis are larger than the epidermal collections of tumour cells, and mitoses may be present in the dermal component. The presence of mitoses and the larger groups of cells in the papillary dermis imply that proliferation of the atypical melanocytes has occurred in the dermis itself, and for this reason any mitotic activity at all in the dermis is considered diagnostic of the vertical growth phase. When invasive tumour fills and expands the papillary dermis (level 3) or invades the reticular dermis (level 4) or the subcutaneous fat (level 5), vertical growth, ipso facto, is present. These tumours are frequently asymmetrical and have poorly defined lateral limits, where single atypical melanocytes and irregular clusters of cells may extend well beyond the invasive component at the dermo-epidermal junction and in a pagetoid pattern within the epidermis. In many cases, a melanocytic naevus co-exists with the melanoma, frequently presenting a nested junctional pattern with or without features of melanocytic dysplasia and with or without a dermal component. Ulceration is seen more commonly in larger tumours, especially those in which an expansile nodule of dermal invasion has developed. Partial regression may be present, manifested by zones of cellular fibrosis, increased vascularity, melanophages and absence of melanoma cells in a segment of epidermis and underlying dermis with tumour adjacent to or on both sides of this altered zone. A lymphocytic stromal reaction is frequently present, especially in association with the less deeply invasive tumours, either at the periphery of the tumour itself or infiltrating the invasive melanoma (tumour-infiltrating lymphocytes). In contrast to dermal melanocytic naevi, cells of superficial spreading melanoma tend to show little or no evidence of maturation in the deeper layers, where the cells retain the same size and other morphological features of those in the superficial layers, and the growth pattern is either expansile or infiltrative, with areas of necrosis in the larger nodules of invasive tumour.

Although the invasive component of superficial spreading melanoma is usually composed of large epithelioid melanocytes, these tumours sometimes include other morphological variants including balloon cells, bizarre giant cells and spindle cells. In some cases, the invasive tumour consists of smaller epithelioid melanocytes with scanty cytoplasm, tending to preserve a nested pattern in the deeper layers, suggesting a naevoid growth pattern. In these tumours, however, the collections of cells are of irregular size and shape, and the neoplastic cells, although relatively small, have atypical, hyperchromatic nuclei, usually with mitoses. Dermal mitoses are essentially diagnostic of melanoma in this context; exceptions include certain simulants discussed elsewhere in this volume, especially Spitz naevi and cellular blue naevi. The presence of heavy melanin pigmentation in some tumours necessitates the use of bleaching to reveal the cytological detail.

The smallest tumours, which may be only 2–3 mm in diameter, are observed as flat or very slightly elevated pigmented lesions with irregular borders. However, most lesions are much larger than this (more than 6 mm at diagnosis). Most lesions are elevated, forming a plaque which is classically asymmetrical with an irregular border and varied pigmentation, ranging from only a few millimetres to several centimetres in diameter. Development of a deeply invasive tumour usually produces an elevated nodule, which may become ulcerated.

1.2.2 Lentigo maligna (Fig. 22)

1.2.3 Lentigo maligna melanoma (Fig. 23)

Lentigo maligna (Hutchinson melanotic freckle) is a linear proliferation of atypical melanocytes along the basal layer of atrophic epidermis and appendages in sun-exposed skin. In lentigo maligna melanoma, in addition to the changes of lentigo maligna, there is dermal invasion by atypical melanocytes.

Lentigo maligna is characterized by the presence of increased numbers of atypical melanocytes in a linear pattern along the dermo-epidermal junction of atrophic epidermis, overlying severe solar elastosis. The neoplastic cells show pronounced nuclear pleomorphism and hyperchromatism and are often composed mainly of spindle-shaped cells with varied pigmentation. Irregular nests of these cells also form at the dermo-epidermal junction, particularly in the larger tumours, and infiltration of the upper layers of the epidermis by single tumour cells may also be present. The atypical melanocytic proliferation also involves the walls of hair follicles and sweat ducts and is usually associated with a patchy lymphocytic infiltrate and scattered melanophages in the superficial dermis. When dermal invasion occurs, the invasive cells are frequently spindle cells, but epithelioid cells and tumour giant cells may also be found. The degree of pigmentation varies, including cells with abundant clear cytoplasm adjacent to cells in which morphological detail may be obscured by coarse granules of melanin. The vertical growth phase in lentigo maligna melanoma may be desmoplastic and/or *neurotropic*; these possibilities should always be considered in evaluating specimen margins.

Lentigo maligna (Hutchinson melanotic freckle), in its classical presentation, appears as a large, flat, variably pigmented patch with irregular borders on the faces of elderly persons. The tumour may occur on any chronically sun-exposed site, however, and much smaller lesions, sometimes only a few millimetres in diameter, are now being diagnosed. The presence of dermal invasion produces clinically apparent plaques or nodules. Lentigo maligna melanoma is much less commonly associated with melanocytic naevi than superficial spreading melanoma.

1.2.4 Nodular melanoma (Fig. 24)

A malignant tumour of epidermal melanocytes without an adjacent epidermal component of in situ melanoma, i.e. without evidence of a pre-existing non-tumorigenic or radial growth phase.

Nodular melanoma is composed of an expansile and infiltrating mass of atypical, variably pigmented melanocytes, usually elevating the epidermis to produce a dome-shaped tumour which is often ulcerated. Atypical melanocytic proliferation is usually present at the overlying dermo-epidermal junction in nested and/or linear patterns, frequently with pagetoid infiltration of the epidermis, as seen in superficial spreading melanoma, but without extension into the adjacent epidermis, the feature which distinguishes between these two types of melanoma. The cells are most often of epithelioid type, but some tumours also contain spindle cells, giant cells or balloon cells. Nuclear pleomorphism is frequently pronounced, with large nucleoli and plentiful mitoses. Several morphologically quite distinct cell populations may be present in the same tumour, and the degree of pigmentation is frequently varied within the one tumour; many nodular melanomas are amelanotic or show only sparse pigmentation in scattered cells. An associated benign melanocytic naevus, sometimes with features of dysplasia, may be present, although less frequently than in association with superficial spreading melanoma.

Nodular melanoma, by definition, is always in the tumorigenic or vertical growth phase at the time of diagnosis, having invaded at least to the papillary–reticular dermal interface and usually into the reticular dermis or subcutis. A patchy lymphocytic reaction may be present in the stroma of the tumour and in the adjacent dermis, but lymphocytes are usually very sparse or absent in the deeper layers of the tumour.

Nodular melanoma occurs on all cutaneous surfaces, presenting a nodular, polypoid or plaque-like protruding mass, frequently ulcerated, with varied pigmentation, including non-pigmented tumours and various shades of brown with pink or violaceous areas in some cases and entirely black tumours, ranging from less than 10 mm to several centimetres in diameter.

1.2.5 Melanoma with unclassified epidermal component

Some melanomas, usually small lesions, have an adjacent epidermal component of atypical melanocytic proliferation in a pattern of neither the classical superficial spreading nor the lentigo maligna type, sometimes showing features of both. These lesions do not fit precisely into either category and may be termed unclassified melanoma (i.e. melanoma with an unclassified epidermal component).

1.2.6 Acral-lentiginous melanoma (Fig. 25)

A melanoma of acral skin with an intra-epidermal component of atypical melanocytes in a lentiginous pattern.

The epidermis is hyperplastic, often with hyperkeratosis. Atypical melanocytes are arranged in a subtle, intermittent linear pattern along the dermo-epidermal junction at the edges of the lesion, becoming more confluent and prominent towards the centre, where atypical cells may also be seen in the lower layers of the epidermis. A typical pagetoid pattern may also be present in the centre of the tumour, indistinguishable from that of superficial spreading melanoma. Some heavily pigmented atypical melanocytes have very prominent, long dendritic processes. The invasive component is composed of either plump spindle or epithelioid cells; a lichenoid lymphocytic infiltrate is characteristic of these tumours and may often obscure the junctional melanocytic proliferation. Invasive spindle cells are often arranged in a neuroid pattern and may demonstrate neurotropism.

The main value of this classification lies in the epidemiological features of these melanomas, which occur with approximately equal frequency in people of all races. In Japan, for instance, acral-lentiginous melanoma is the most common form, although the population-based incidence of all types of melanoma is low. Co-existent naevi and evidence of actinic damage are seldom seen in association with these tumours. Acral-lentiginous melanomas occur most frequently on the volar skin of the feet and on the palms. Subungual melanoma, a subset of acral-lentiginous melanoma, occurs most commonly on the thumb and great toe.

1.2.7 Mucosal-lentiginous melanoma

A melanoma of mucosal surfaces with an adjacent intramucosal component of lentiginous pattern.

Atypical melanocytes, often with prominent dendrites, are arranged in a lentiginous pattern along the basal layer of the epithelium, often with an associated lichenoid infiltrate and areas of regression. A few atypical melanocytes are also usually seen above the basal layer, but pagetoid infiltration of the epithelium is rare. The invasive component is often of spindle cell type with desmoplastic and neurotropic features.

The plaque or radial growth phase of mucosal-lentiginous melanoma shows varied pigmentation, including amelanotic areas, and the borders are frequently ill defined. Tumorigenic or vertical growth phase often presents as an ulcerated globoid mass. The most common sites are the vulva, vagina, oral cavity and nasal sinuses. Tumours of the anal canal, oesophagus and urethra are less common.

1.2.8 Desmoplastic melanoma (Fig. 26)

A spindle cell melanoma, usually diagnosed in the tumorigenic or vertical growth phase, associated with desmoplasia and, frequently, neuroid differentiation and neurotropism.

Most of these tumours have an intra-epidermal component, although often relatively inconspicuous and of limited extent, usually in a lentiginous pattern of the lentigo maligna type. Nested junctional and pagetoid intra-epidermal proliferation of epithelioid melanocytes may also be present, although less commonly. In some cases the invasive cells are of spindle cell type throughout the tumour, including the papillary dermis, whereas in other cases the invasive cells in the superficial dermis are of epithelioid type, gradually blending with spindle cells in the deeper layers. In some cases, however, no intra-epidermal component is found. The dermal component is of varied cellularity, composed of spindle cells separated by slender collagen bundles, presenting a relatively bland appearance at low power. Individual tumour cells may be widely separated by thick bundles of sclerotic collagen extending into the subcutis where infiltration may be inconspicuous. Other lesions are more densely cellular, with plump spindle cells arranged in broad fascicles, some of which may be arranged vertically, separated by relatively sparse collagenous stroma. A prominent, patchy infiltrate of lymphocytes is a characteristic feature in the stroma. The degree of cytological atypia varies between different tumours and between zones of the same tumour, ranging from minimal atypia in uniform spindle cells to markedly atypical cells with pleomorphic nuclei, large nucleoli and numerous mitoses. Infiltration of the perineurium and endoneurium is recognized by the presence of atypical nuclei, sometimes with a lymphocytic infiltrate in the adjacent stroma. The stroma may contain myxoid areas with abundant mucin, whereas in other areas a pattern resembling neurofibroma may be seen, where the atypical spindle cells are embedded in wavy bundles of collagen fibres. These neoplasms, which often contain little or no melanin, may be misdiagnosed as neural or fibrohistiocytic tumours, benign or malignant, but the range of possible misdiagnoses is extremely broad and varied. Immunostaining for S100 protein and vimentin is usually positive, but staining for HMB45 is often negative.

Desmoplastic melanomas occur most commonly on the exposed skin. As they are frequently amelanotic or only very lightly pigmented with poorly defined borders, often flat or only slightly elevated, these tumours are frequently misdiagnosed clinically as well as histologically, posing one of the most difficult diagnostic problems in cutaneous neoplasms.

1.2.9 Neurotropic melanoma

A melanoma that invades nerves; most of these tumours are spindle cell melanomas and many are desmoplastic, but neurotropism can occur in any histological type of melanoma.

Apart from the more common histological variants of melanoma and desmoplastic melanoma that may exhibit neurotropism, some neurotropic melanomas, besides invading the perineural space and the endoneurium, also show apparent neuroid differentiation in areas where the spindle-shaped tumour cells have serpiginous nuclei and are embedded in a fibrillar stroma.

Another category of neurotropic spindle cell neoplasm is the *superficial malignant epithelioid schwannoma*, which is probably synonymous with "nerve-centred desmoplastic melanoma", characterized by the presence of neoplastic spindle cells in structures resembling nerve fascicles and expanded nerve trunks. These terms should be reserved for neurotropic spindle cell neoplasms without pigment or an epidermal component of atypical melanocytes. The term "pigmented superficial malignant epithelioid schwannoma" is probably best regarded as synonymous with "neurotropic melanoma".

The clinical features are similar to those of desmoplastic melanoma.

1.2.10 Malignant blue naevus (Fig. 27)

A malignant dermal melanocytic neoplasm associated with a benign blue naevus, usually of cellular type.

The epidermis is usually not involved, overlying a nodular, densely cellular, predominantly spindle cell tumour including heavily pigmented cells, usually extending into the deep dermis or subcutis. The tumour includes areas indistinguishable from common blue naevus or cellular blue naevus, but features suggesting malignancy are the greater size of the tumour, denser cellularity and presence of necrosis. The growth pattern is fascicular, without the characteristic biphasic pattern of cellular blue naevus. Mitoses are usually present, but not plentiful.

Although so-called benign metastases from blue naevus have been well documented, consisting of small groups of cells only in the peripheral sinus of lymph nodes, the metastases from malignant blue naevi replace the lymph node parenchyma, and the metastatic cells show severe cytological atypia and more frequent mitoses, including atypical forms.

Malignant blue naevi are extremely rare. The tumours are blue or bluish-black nodules, usually greater than 3 cm in diameter and sometimes multinodular. The most common site is the scalp. Most cases appear to have developed in a pre-existing cellular blue naevus which may have been present for many years before metastasis occurs.

1.2.11 Melanoma in congenital melanocytic naevi (Figs. 28, 29)

The incidence of malignant change in small and intermediate congenital naevi is low, and the congenital naevus-associated melanoma usually occurs in adult life and is of the superficial spreading type. Melanoma in giant congenital naevi has been reported to occur in 4.6%–10% of cases. Melanomas may occur in giant congenital naevi during childhood, sometimes entirely within the dermal component of the naevus, where they may include an unusual variety of cell types and growth patterns, including atypical spindle and/or epithelioid cells with necrosis, infiltrative growth and mitoses. Heterotopic elements such as striated muscle and cartilage may be present. Small cell variants are composed of masses of atypical cells with scanty cytoplasm and hyperchromatic nuclei presenting a blastomatous appearance. In adult life, melanomas developing in giant naevi tend to be of the superficial spreading type, as is also the case in most melanomas associated with small congenital naevi.

1.2.12 Minimal deviation melanoma (Fig. 30)

A melanoma in vertical (tumorigenic) growth phase, composed of cells that are less atypical than those of the common forms of melanoma. The concept of minimal-deviation melanoma has not been universally accepted.

Melanocytic tumours included in this category are composed of nodules with expansile intradermal growth and very little, if any, adjacent intra-epidermal component. The tumours are relatively monomorphous, the predominant cell types being spindle cells and small epithelioid or nevoid cells. Some tumours show Spitzoid features.

Minimal deviation melanoma has been reported to occur in childhood and adult life, with an equal sex ratio. Some lesions have presented clinical features suggestive of Spitz naevus or haemangioma. The prognosis of lesions diagnosed as minimal deviation melanomas is relatively good.

1.2.13 Clear cell sarcoma[1]

1.2.14 Malignant melanocytic schwannoma[1]

1.3 Non-neoplastic hyperpigmentations

1.3.1 Ephelis (freckle)

A small pigmented macule characterized by increased melanogenesis without proliferation of epidermal melanocytes.

The epidermis shows normal architecture and hyperpigmentation of melanocytes, which are present in normal number.

---

[1] Defined as in Weiss SW (1994) Histological typing of soft tissue tumours, WHO International Histological Classification of Tumours. Springer-Verlag, Berlin Heidelberg New York.

Freckles occur on the sun-exposed skin of children and adults with fair complexions.

1.3.2 Solar (actinic) lentigo

An irregular, poorly circumscribed pigmented macule of actinically damaged skin.

The epidermis is slightly hyperplastic with variable elongation of rete ridges, hyperpigmentation of the basal layer and normal or slightly increased number of melanocytes. Solar elastosis and melanophages are present in the dermis.

Variably pigmented patches range from a few millimetres to more than 1 cm in diameter, of varied shape with poorly defined borders. Their frequency increases with age on the exposed skin of individuals with fair complexions.

1.3.3 Mucosal melanosis (genital lentiginosis)

A benign, flat, pigmented macular lesion of mucosal epithelium and adjacent skin.

The basal layer is hyperpigmented with mild keratinocytic hyperplasia, melanocytes in normal or slightly increased number and melanophages in the superficial stroma.

These irregular, often deeply pigmented lesions, especially on the vulva, may simulate melanoma. Similar lesions of the lip are usually smaller and less pigmented.

1.3.4 Café au lait spot

A congenital or acquired macular lesion of uniform pale pigmentation and variable size.

Melanin pigmentation of keratinocytes is slightly increased in epidermis of normal architecture. The number of melanocytes is normal, but giant melanosomes may be present.

Solitary café au lait spots are common; multiple lesions are usually associated with von Recklinghausen neurofibromatosis.

TNM Classification (Staging System) for Melanoma[1]

The TNM system of tumour staging considers factors related to the primary tumour, to regional lymph nodes and to distant

---

[1] Hermanek P, Sobin LH (eds) (1992) TNM Classification of Malignant Tumours, 4th edn (2nd revision). Springer-Verlag, Berlin Heidelberg New York.

metastases to result in a classification that is associated with the probability of survival. In the current system, the T attributes are classified pathologically after excision of the melanoma (pT) as follows:

pT – Primary Tumour

- pTX Primary tumour cannot be assessed
- pT0 No evidence of primary tumour
- pTis Melanoma in situ (Clark level I) (atypical melanocytic hyperplasia, severe melanocytic dysplasia, not an invasive malignant lesion)
- pT1 Tumour 0.75 mm or less in thickness invading the papillary dermis (Clark level II)
- pT2 Tumour more than 0.75 mm, but not more than 1.5 mm in thickness and/or invading as far as the papillary–reticular dermal interface (Clark level III)
- pT3 Tumour more than 1.5 mm, but not more than 4.0 mm in thickness and/or invading the reticular dermis (Clark level IV)
  - pT3a Tumour more than 1.5 mm, but not more than 3.0 mm in thickness
  - pT3b Tumour more than 3.0 mm, but not more than 4.0 mm in thickness
- pT4 Tumour more than 4.0 mm in thickness and/or invading the subcutaneous tissue (Clark level V) and/or satellites within 2 cm of the primary tumour
  - pT4a Tumour more than 4.0 mm in thickness and/or invading the subcutaneous tissue
  - pT4b Satellite(s) within 2 cm of the primary tumour

N – Regional Lymph Nodes (Clinical Staging)

- NX Regional lymph nodes cannot be assessed
- N0 No regional lymph node metastasis
- N1 Metastasis 3 cm or less in greatest dimension in any regional lymph node(s)
- N2 Metastasis more than 3 cm in greatest dimension in any regional lymph node(s) and/or in transit metastasis
  - N2a Metastasis more than 3 cm in greatest dimension in any regional lymph node(s)
  - N2b In transit metastasis
  - N2c Both

Note: In transit metastasis involves skin or subcutaneous tissue more than 2 cm from the primary tumour, but not beyond the regional lymph nodes.

M – Distant metastasis

MX Presence of distant metastasis cannot be assessed
M0 No distant metastasis
M1 Distant metastasis
  M1a Metastasis in skin or subcutaneous tissue or lymph node(s) beyond the regional lymph nodes
  M1b Visceral metastasis
pN Categories correspond to the N categories
pM Categories correspond to the M categories

Stage Grouping

Stage I	pT1	N0	M0
	pT2	N0	M0
Stage II	pT3	N0	M0
Stage III	pT4	N0	M0
	Any pT	N1, N2	M0
Stage IV	Any pT	Any N	M1

Tumours in stages I and II are non-metastatic, and stage III may or not be associated with metastasis. Since these stages are different from those defined in other commonly used staging systems, it is clear that the system in use should be clearly specified when a staging classification is used as a basis for therapy or prognosis. The TNM system described above explicitly equates levels of invasion with particular thickness ranges, which may be appropriate when each is considered as a single variable. However, thickness is more powerfully predictive of survival when evaluated in multivariate models, and if a single variable is to be considered as the major predictor of survival, it should be thickness. The TNM model considers pathological attributes of the primary tumour, but staging for lymph node metastases is defined both clinically and pathologically in terms of the diameter of the largest metastasis. In patients with regional lymph node metastases, survival has also been correlated with the number of lymph nodes involved and the tumour volume.

2 Epidermal Tumours

2.1 Benign

2.1.1 Epidermal

2.1.1.1 Epidermal naevus (Fig. 31)

A benign papillomatous epidermal tumour, either congenital or becoming clinically apparent early in life.

These are epidermal proliferations with hyperkeratosis, mild acanthosis and papillomatosis, sometimes resembling seborrhoeic keratosis.

Epidermal naevi occur as linear keratotic plaques or papules of varied size on the trunk or limbs.

2.1.1.2 Seborrhoeic keratosis (Fig. 32)

An exophytic tumour composed of acanthotic, papillomatous epidermis and interlocking downgrowths of uniform basaloid cells, with invaginations forming horn cysts.

These lesions are sharply demarcated and frequently polypoid. Variable pigmentation is present in the basaloid cells, and foci of hyperkeratosis at the surface may be continuous with keratin-filled invaginations pushing into the body of the tumour, whereas other horn cysts apparently have no connection with the surface. The cells surrounding the horn cysts show more squamoid differentiation, including granular cells and prickle cells.

Variants

Irritated seborrhoeic keratosis. Irritation of seborrhoeic keratosis, expressed by the presence of lymphocytic inflammation in the superficial dermis and in the body of the neoplasm, is associated with more pronounced squamous differentiation and the presence of squamoid eddies.

Adenoid or reticulated seborrhoeic keratosis. This tumour consists of interlocking, slender cords of basaloid cells, frequently pigmented, forming a network including keratin cysts.

Plane seborrhoeic keratosis. These lesions are only slightly elevated and are frequently heavily pigmented.

Seborrhoeic keratosis with an intra-epidermal epithelioma pattern (clonal seborrhoeic keratosis). Seborrhoeic keratoses may include an intra-epidermal epithelioma pattern of growth (Borst-Jadassohn phenomenon) with formation of well-defined nests of small, uniform basaloid cells within the epidermis sharply demarcated from the adjacent normal keratinocytes. This is not a distinctive lesion.

Melanoacanthoma. A rare variant in which pigmented melanocytes are present in association with relatively amelanotic neoplastic basaloid cells.

Inverted follicular keratosis (Fig. 33). This lesion, characterized by a more inverted growth pattern, is apparently produced by involvement of follicular epithelium by the seborrhoeic keratosis. These tumours include blunt downgrowths of basaloid epithelium and numerous small squamoid eddies.

Benign squamous keratosis (keratotic papilloma). In these small lesions, the epidermal proliferation consists of mature keratinocytes rather than basaloid cells, with only occasional horn cysts.

Clinical features. Seborrhoeic keratoses are extremely common lesions that occur on the trunk, arms and face, mainly in middle-aged or elderly people, sometimes as multiple lesions. The tumours have a verrucous, plaque-like or polypoid appearance of uniform tan to dark brown or black colour with a velvety or granular surface.

2.1.1.3 Clear cell acanthoma (Fig. 34)

A benign neoplasm of squamoid keratinocytes containing abundant cytoplasmic glycogen.

The tumour consists of intra-epidermal aggregates of keratinocytes with clear cytoplasm forming blunt downgrowths with elongation of the rete ridges, sharply demarcated from the adjacent normal epidermal cells. Parakeratosis overlies the tumour, which is often infiltrated by neutrophils.

These uncommon lesions occur as pale, slightly elevated, frequently ulcerated lesions on the legs of middle-aged and elderly individuals.

2.1.1.4 Fibroepithelial polyp (skin tag, acrochordon) (Fig. 35)

Sessile or pedunculated soft, flesh-coloured, benign epithelial tumours with a fibrovascular core.

The epidermis is raised in a polypoid pattern overlying a fibrovascular core in which mature adipose tissue and nerve fibres may also proliferate.

These are common lesions typically on the trunk, head and neck of elderly people.

2.1.1.5 Warty dyskeratoma (isolated dyskeratosis follicularis) (Fig. 36)

A solitary epidermal neoplasm characterized by acantholysis and dyskeratosis of the squamous epithelial wall surrounding a crater-like depression containing keratin.

Endophytic downgrowths of squamous epithelium form the wall of a crater-like invagination filled with laminated keratin. Acantholytic dyskeratotic cells including corps ronds, grains and suprabasal clefts overlie papillary protrusions of dermis covered by a single layer of basal cells, presenting a villous pattern.

Warty dyskeratoma is usually an isolated tumour on the scalp, face or neck.

2.1.1.6 Actinic keratosis (solar keratosis) (Figs. 37, 38)

A premalignant, i.e. potentially malignant, lesion characterized by localized intra-epidermal keratinocytic atypia in sun-damaged skin.

In early lesions, small mounds of parakeratosis overlie slightly acanthotic epidermis in which the cells of the basal and lower spinous layers are atypical, with dyskeratosis and enlarged nuclei. Small, blunt downgrowths of these cells push into the superficial dermis without frank infiltration of the stroma, associated with a patchy lymphocytic infiltrate and elastosis. Thicker columns of parakeratosis and sometimes prominent cutaneous horns overlie the larger lesions of actinic keratosis. In some lesions, full-thickness squamous cell atypia (in situ squamous cell carcinoma) develops, followed, again in only a proportion of cases, by dermal invasion (squamous cell carcinoma). Acantholysis is prominent in some lesions. The adjacent epidermis is frequently atrophic, whereas the involved epidermis may be thickened or atrophic. The squamous epithelium in the walls of acrosyringia is frequently preserved intact without cellular atypia in zones of actinic keratosis. Variants include *hyperplastic actinic keratosis (proliferative actinic keratosis), lichenoid actinic keratosis* with a dense lymphocytic infiltrate in the superficial dermis and *large cell acanthoma* characterized by minimal atypia and well-demarcated proliferation of pale, enlarged keratinocytes.

Actinic keratoses occur as small (less than 10mm in diameter), often multiple, scaly erythematous lesions, sometimes with cutaneous horn formation, on the sun-exposed skin of fair-skinned people, most commonly in the elderly but also in young adults who are habitually exposed to strong sunlight.

2.1.1.7 Keratoacanthoma (Fig. 39)

An exophytic epidermal neoplasm containing a central keratin-filled crater-like depression.

Keratoacanthoma has a distinctive architecture, presenting protuberant squamous epithelium forming the walls of a central crater-like depression filled with keratin and extending down into the dermis, sometimes almost to the subcutis. Blunt downgrowths of squamous epithelium extend into the dermis without true infiltration of the stroma, presenting an irregular lower border. Cellular fibrosis and a mixed inflammatory infiltrate, often including neutrophils, are present at the edges of the tumour; groups of neutrophils ("microabscesses") are also seen within the body of the tumour. Keratoacanthomas are composed mainly of large squamous cells with pale eosinophilic or clear cytoplasm containing abundant glycogen. The cells at the periphery of the tumour lobules are of more basaloid type. Moderate nuclear pleomorphism and mitoses may be seen, but atypical mitotic figures and stromal infiltration suggest the diagnosis of well-differentiated squamous cell carcinoma. Regressing lesions tend to become more superficial with a flattened base, more mature, uniform epithelium and denser fibrosis in the surrounding stroma.

The histological distinction of keratoacanthoma from well-differentiated squamous cell carcinoma may be difficult, in accordance with the theory that keratoacanthoma represents a variant of carcinoma characterized by rapid growth and involution. Tumours with the classical architectural features of keratoacanthoma which also show dermal invasion by atypical squamous cells should be classified as well-differentiated squamous cell carcinoma.

Keratoacanthomas occur mainly on the exposed skin of the face and the dorsa of the hands. Rapid growth produces a crater-like lesion with a central keratin plug, becoming flattened during the slow process of spontaneous regression. Variants include the following:

- *Giant keratoacanthoma*
- *Keratoacanthoma centrifugum marginatum*, which undergoes progressive growth by peripheral extension
- *Subungual keratoacanthoma*, a destructive form that may produce erosion of the terminal phalanx
- *Multiple keratoacanthomas* in association with immunosuppression and with Torre syndrome
- *Multiple eruptive keratoacanthomas* (multiple self-healing epitheliomas of the Ferguson-Smith type), which develop in children and adolescents on any cutaneous surface

2.1.1.8 Benign lichenoid keratosis (lichen planus-like keratosis) (Fig. 40)

A solitary benign epidermal lesion associated with severe lichenoid inflammation.

The epidermis is usually slightly hyperplastic, with focal parakeratosis, and basal layer degeneration overlying a lichenoid lymphocytic infiltrate. The lesions are small (3–10mm), usually solitary and often associated with an adjacent solar lentigo. Lichenoid keratosis should not be confused with lichenoid actinic keratosis, in which there is cellular atypia.

Lichenoid keratosis occurs as a violaceous papule in adults and probably represents a cell-mediated reaction to a variety of benign lesions such as solar lentigo.

2.1.2 Verrucae (virus-related lesions)

Benign squamous papillomatous neoplasms caused by human papilloma virus infection. Subtypes include verruca vulgaris (common wart), verruca plantaris (plantar wart), verruca plana (flat wart) and condyloma acuminatum.

2.1.2.1 Verruca vulgaris (common wart) (Fig. 41)

Verruca vulgaris is characterized by outgrowths of epidermis presenting slender spires, as in filiform wart, or blunter digitate processes, as in the common wart. The squamous epithelium is acanthotic with hyperkeratosis and columns of parakeratosis at the apices of the projections. Hypergranulosis is prominent where enlarged, rounded keratohyaline granules are present. Koilocytic change with cytoplasmic clearing and pyknotic nuclei is seen in cells in the upper stratum malpighii and granular layer. A very characteristic dispersion of chromatin may be seen in affected nuclei in the upper epidermal layers, resulting in a steel-grey pallor. Eosinophilic granular inclusions may also be seen in these zones of pallor. The dermal stroma contains dilated, tortuous blood vessels. Elongated rete ridges at the lateral margins of the tumour slant inwards towards the centre.

These extremely common hyperkeratotic lesions occur most frequently on the fingers and on the dorsum of the hand, but also on any cutaneous surface.

2.1.2.2 Verruca plantaris (plantar wart) (Fig. 42)

These tumours, characterized by a less exophytic architecture than verruca vulgaris, are composed of broad, irregular downgrowths of squamous epithelium below a mound of hyperkeratosis and parakeratosis. Large, irregular eosinophilic cytoplasmic inclusions are frequently seen in the upper layers of the epidermis.

Plantar warts are solitary or multiple, poorly defined lesions on the sole.

2.1.2.3 Verruca plana (flat wart) (Fig. 43)

These tumours are slightly raised, flat papules. Hyperkeratosis and acanthosis are present, but the pronounced papillomatosis and parakeratosis of verruca vulgaris are absent. The upper layers of the epidermis contain plentiful vacuolated keratinocytes, and the stratum corneum has a prominent basket-weave appearance.

Flat warts occur as multiple, flesh-coloured papules, often in a linear distribution, usually on the hands and feet.

2.1.2.4 Condyloma acuminatum (Fig. 44)

A verruca occurring on the genitalia or anal region.

Condylomata acuminata show exophytic and endophytic proliferation of squamous epithelium with pronounced acanthosis, papillomatosis and parakeratosis. Keratinocytes with perinuclear vacuolization and pyknotic, hyperchromatic "wrinkled" nuclei (koilocytes) are present in the upper layers. Scattered dyskeratotic and apoptotic keratinocytes may be present in the upper layers of the epidermis.

Condylomata acuminata, induced by human papillomavirus (HPV) infection, usually HPV-6, occur most commonly on the genitalia and less frequently in the perianal region and anal canal. They are often multiple and cover large areas of skin and mucosa. Although usually exophytic, pink or white warty tumours, flat papules and pigmented variants also occur. Simple condyloma acuminatum, giant condyloma acuminatum and verrucous carcinoma may constitute a continuous but not obligatory spectrum of developing malignancy.

2.1.2.5 Giant condyloma acuminatum (Buschke and Lowenstein)

A very large variant of condyloma acuminatum.

Giant condyloma acuminatum shows the same changes as condyloma acuminatum on an exaggerated scale, with a greatly thickened stratum corneum and deep, expansile growths of acanthotic epithelium. The extreme degree of endophytic epithelial growth mimics pseudoepitheliomatous hyperplasia or true invasion.

These tumours are similar in their architecture and morphology to condyloma acuminatum, but they are much larger, often cauliflower-like and ulcerated, usually single, occurring most commonly on the prepuce of the penis, forming fungating and destructive, but non-invasive growths. A few cases have been reported in the perianal and ano-rectal regions. Giant condylomata grow slowly and tend to recur, eventually infiltrating the soft tissues causing sinuses and fistulae.

2.1.2.6 Bowenoid papulosis (Fig. 45)

A small, papular epidermal tumour associated with HPV-16 infection characterized by atypical squamous cells scattered among orderly squamous epithelium.

The tumours are sharply circumscribed, exophytic epidermal proliferations with irregular acanthosis, hyperkeratosis and parakeratosis. Atypical squamous cells are scattered throughout the epidermis in a "salt and pepper" arrangement against a background of orderly, stratified epithelium, in contrast with Bowen disease, in which the atypical cells are confluent and occupy the full thickness of the epidermis with complete distortion of stratification. Koilocytes are sometimes present, but they are not as prominent as in condyloma acuminatum.

Bowenoid papulosis occurs as single or multiple, small (average size, 4mm), reddish-brown papules, sometimes forming plaques with a verrucoid appearance, mainly on the glans, foreskin and shaft of the penis in young men and in the perineal and vulvar areas in women.

2.1.2.7 Molluscum contagiosum (Fig. 46)

A lesion composed of inverted lobules of squamous epithelium expanding into the underlying dermis and containing characteristic cytoplasmic inclusion bodies.

The lobules of squamous epithelium contain eosinophilic inclusion bodies, appearing above the basal layer and enlarging progressively in the upper layers, where the inclusions become increasingly basophilic, occupying the entire cell in the granular layer. Molluscum bodies are extruded with keratinous debris into ostia leading to the epidermis.

The lesions present as solitary or multiple, well-circumscribed, dome-shaped, umbilicated papules, often on the flexor areas or genitalia of children and young adults. The molluscum bodies contain a DNA pox virus.

2.2 Malignant

2.2.1 Squamous cell carcinoma (Figs. 47, 48)

A malignant neoplasm of epidermis showing evidence of squamous cell differentiation.

In situ squamous cell carcinoma. Atypia of keratinocytes at all levels of the epidermis produces distortion of stratification, usually in association with thickening of the epidermis and parakeratosis. The cellular atypia may be of moderate degree in some cases, whereas in others nuclear pleomorphism and hyperchromatism are pronounced, including giant forms and plentiful mitoses. The in situ carcinoma may be associated with adjacent solar keratosis or, in unexposed sites, sharply demarcated from normal epidermis, as in the Bowen disease variant of in situ squamous cell carcinoma.

Invasive squamous cell carcinoma. Invasive squamous cell carcinoma in exposed skin occurs often, but not invariably, in association with actinic keratosis, with or without in situ carcinoma. The invasive tumour may be well differentiated, composed of sheets and strands of cells displaying prominent intercellular bridges and central keratin pearls. In poorly differentiated tumours, pronounced nuclear pleomorphism and hyperchromatism are present, and giant forms may be seen; nucleoli are large and mitoses plentiful.

Variants

2.2.1.1 Spindle cell squamous cell carcinoma (Fig. 49)

An uncommon form composed of elongated cells arranged in sheets and in a diffuse pattern in a fibroblastic stroma.

2.2.1.2 Acantholytic squamous cell carcinoma

Acantholysis of tumour cells produces a pseudoglandular pattern.

2.2.1.3 Verrucous squamous cell carcinoma (Fig. 50)

A well-differentiated squamous cell carcinoma with minimal cellular atypia, keratotic papillary spikes and a blunt, pushing deep border. According to different authorities, verrucous carcinoma has been regarded as a separate entity or as identical to giant condyloma.

The only microscopic distinction, if any, between verrucous squamous cell carcinoma and giant condyloma is the presence of true invasion in the carcinomatous lesion. The blunt downgrowths of squamous epithelium are well differentiated, often lacking atypia, but moderate nuclear pleomorphism and mitotic activity may be present.

Verrucous squamous cell carcinomas are tumours of the oral mucosa, the genitalia, perianal region and the anal canal, where they form large cauliflower-like tumours, similar to giant condyloma acuminatum, and also of the soles, palms and other cutaneous sites, with the potential for metastasis in rare cases usually after an indolent course. Those tumours of the sole characterized by deeply invasive interlocking branches of squamous cells forming tunnels and clefts have also been termed *epithelioma cuniculatum.*

2.2.1.4 Squamous cell carcinoma with horn formation

Keratotic horns may arise from both in situ and invasive squamous cell carcinoma.

2.2.1.5 Lymphoepithelial squamous cell carcinoma (Fig. 51)

A rare variant resembling nasopharyngeal lymphoepithelial carcinoma, composed of poorly differentiated cords and islands of invasive tumour cells embedded in a dense lymphocytic infiltrate. The absence of connection with the epidermis and the occasional presence of intracytoplasmic mucin in tumour cells suggest that this may be a poorly differentiated adnexal carcinoma rather than a true squamous cell carcinoma.

Squamous cell carcinomas occur mainly on sun-exposed skin of elderly people, but they can occur on all cutaneous surfaces and in younger patients, especially those with fair complexions. These tumours present as hyperkeratotic, sometimes ulcerated, indurated plaques or nodules. Some well-differentiated squamous cell carcinomas have a prominent, nodular shape with a central crater-like depression, similar to keratoacanthoma. Ultraviolet light is the most important aetiological factor in the commonest form of squamous cell carcinoma arising in solar keratosis, but other aetiological factors include previous burns, chronic inflammation, immunosuppression, industrial carcinogens, chronic ulcers and osteomyelitis, ionizing radiation and xeroderma pigmentosum, a defect in DNA repair associated with a high incidence of squamous cell carcinoma. Squamous cell carcinomas arising in sun-damaged skin rarely metastasize, whereas metastasis is more common from those tumours related to aetiological factors other than ultraviolet light.

In situ squamous cell carcinoma occurring in unexposed sites (Bowen disease) has been correlated in the past with an increased incidence of internal malignancy, but more recently this association has been questioned.

2.2.2 Basal cell carcinoma

A low-grade malignant epithelial neoplasm composed of cells simulating the basal cell layer of the epidermis.

Many histological variants of basal cell carcinoma occur. The diagnostic features common to all types are groups of basaloid cells with scanty, pale cytoplasm, round or ovoid nuclei and coarse, granular chromatin. The peripheral layer of cells is characteristically arranged in a palisaded pattern, and the surrounding stroma is frequently separated from the tumour by an artefactual cleft. Most tumours are connected with the epidermis and invade the dermis as solid or cystic nodules arranged in various growth patterns. Mitoses may be sparse or plentiful, central necrosis is frequently present, especially in the larger tumour nodules, and intercellular bridges are always present, although less prominent than in squamous cell carcinoma.

Variants

2.2.2.1 Multifocal superficial basal cell carcinoma (superficial multicentric) (Fig. 52)

Multiple small nodules of basaloid cells push down from the epidermis without invading the superficial dermis, sharply demarcated from the adjacent normal epithelium. This multifocal superficial pattern may also be associated with invasive tumour.

2.2.2.2 Nodular basal cell carcinoma (solid, adenoid cystic) (Fig. 53)

This variant, the commonest type of basal cell carcinoma, consists of nodules of varied size with peripheral palisading and retraction artefact, frequently containing central zones of necrosis producing a cystic appearance. An adenoid pattern, composed of thin strands of basaloid cells in a reticulate pattern, may co-exist with the solid and cystic types. The epidermis overlying the tumour is frequently ulcerated, and the surrounding dermal stroma may consist of cellular fibrous tissue or more myxoid, loosely structured stroma.

2.2.2.3 Infiltrating basal cell carcinoma

2.2.2.3.1 Non-sclerosing

In this variant, small groups and strands of basaloid cells infiltrate between the collagen bundles in the deeper dermis, often with a more solid pattern in the superficial layers.

2.2.2.3.2 Sclerosing (desmoplastic, morpheic) (Fig. 54)

Strands and small groups of tumour cells infiltrate the dermis diffusely in a dense, desmoplastic stroma.

2.2.2.4 Fibroepithelial basal cell carcinoma (Fig. 55)

An elevated, nodular tumour composed of interlocking slender strands of basaloid cells in a loose, fibrous stroma.

2.2.2.5 Basal cell carcinoma with adnexal differentiation

2.2.2.5.1 Basal cell carcinoma with follicular differentiation

This tumour is composed of nests of basaloid cells resembling telogen hair follicles, including small keratinous cysts.

2.2.2.5.2 Basal cell carcinoma with eccrine differentiation (Fig. 56)

These tumours are most commonly of nodular pattern, including cystic and adenoid areas. Multiple duct-like structures lined by eosinophilic cuticular epithelium and alveolar groups of tumour cells with vacuolated cytoplasm are present in the tumour islands. These structures may contain epithelial mucin; immunostaining for carcino-embryonic antigen is positive in a linear pattern around the lumina of these structures.

2.2.2.6 Basosquamous carcinoma (Fig. 57)

This controversial variant includes squamoid cells with abundant eosinophilic cytoplasm, smaller, uniform basaloid cells and an intermediate cell with pale cytoplasm of the type described in so-called *metatypical basal cell carcinoma*, which exhibits more severe nuclear pleomorphism and infiltrative growth.

2.2.2.7 Keratotic basal cell carcinoma

These tumours are similar to the common solid basal cell carcinoma, but they also include central foci of more pronounced squamous differentiation with keratinization.

2.2.2.8 Pigmented basal cell carcinoma

Melanin pigmentation is frequently present, mainly in the solid and multifocal superficial types of basal cell carcinoma. Melanocytes are scattered in the tumour islands, with groups of melanophages in the adjacent stroma.

2.2.2.9 Basal cell carcinoma in basal cell naevus syndrome

Multiple basal cell carcinomas, indistinguishable from other basal cell carcinomas, occur in this syndrome in association with cysts of the jaws, bifid ribs and other skeletal and neurological anomalies.

2.2.2.10 Micronodular basal cell carcinoma (Fig. 58)

This variant resembles nodular basal cell carcinoma. The groups of cells, however, are much smaller than those of the common nodular form of basal cell carcinoma, and they tend to invade the dermis deeply, often extending into the subcutis.

Basal cell carcinomas occur most commonly in adults, in densest distribution on the exposed areas of the head and neck, but also on the skin of the trunk and proximal limbs. The incidence is highest in fair-skinned individuals and lowest in black people. In children, they are usually associated with the basal cell naevus syndrome, Basex syndrome, xeroderma pigmentosum or with organoid naevi such as sebaceus naevi. The common nodular type classically has a pearly translucent border with an ulcerated centre (rodent ulcer); multifocal superficial basal cell carcinoma presents as a flat, pale or erythematous, poorly defined patch; the diffusely infiltrating variants are usually flat or slightly depressed, pale, indurated plaques. Metastasis is rare, but local recurrence is more common in the multifocal, infiltrating and micronodular types.

3 Adnexal Tumours

3.1 Eccrine Tumours

3.1.1 Benign

3.1.1.1 Ciliated cyst

A simple cyst lined by ciliated epithelial cells.

The cutaneous cyst is lined by cuboidal or columnar epithelial cells, most of which have prominent cilia. Papillary fibrovascular projections characteristically protrude into the cyst lumen.

These rare tumours occur mainly on the lower extremities of young women.

3.1.1.2 Hidrocystoma (eccrine cystadenoma)

A unilocular cystic nodule resulting from cystic ectasia of the dermal portion of the eccrine duct.

The tumour consists of a large unilocular dilated cyst in the mid-dermis, lined by two layers of cuboidal epithelium, which may be flattened in some areas. Small papillary projections may be present.

Eccrine hidrocystoma is usually a solitary lesion on the face.

3.1.1.3 Papillary eccrine adenoma (Fig. 59)

A rare solitary tumour of eccrine ductal and glandular structures, usually occurring on the hands and feet.

The tumour consists of a circumscribed collection of ductal and glandular structures, some including papillary epithelial projections. The lumina contain amorphous eosinophilic material, but small cysts containing laminated keratin may also be present. The glandular structures are lined by cuboidal epithelium in one or several layers.

The tumours range from 5 to 20 mm in diameter and occur more commonly in black people.

3.1.1.4 Syringoma (Fig. 60)

A benign tumour derived from the eccrine duct, usually multiple, occurring on the face, frequently on the eyelids.

Syringomas are small, usually well-circumscribed tumours composed of small ducts lined by cuboidal or flattened cuticular epithelium, often continuous with a slender solid cord of these cells producing a tadpole- or comma-like contour. In their superficial layers, the tumours frequently include keratotic cysts lined by flattened epithelium. The clear cell variant of syringoma is composed of slightly larger cuboidal cells containing glycogen.

Syringomas are small papular lesions (1–3 mm in diameter), often multiple, but sometimes solitary.

3.1.1.5 Mixed tumour of skin (chondroid syringoma) (Fig. 61)

A tumour of glandular epithelium with myxoid or chondroid stroma.

These are circumscribed, lobular tumours situated in the deep dermis, sometimes extending into the subcutis, composed of glandular structures including ducts lined by a single layer of cuboidal epithelium (eccrine type) or by two rows or more of epithelium, sometimes showing decapitation secretion (apocrine type) and stroma including fibrous, myxoid or chondroid tissue. The varied epithelial component may include solid cords of cuboidal epithelium, small keratotic cysts and groups of cells with clear cytoplasm. The stroma contains acid mucopolysaccharide, spindle cells and rounded cells with plentiful cytoplasm resembling chondrocytes. The origin of the chondroid stroma has been attributed to both the myoepithelial and the epithelial cells. The tumour resembles the pleomorphic adenoma of salivary glands.

These are smooth, firm, nodular tumours of the head and neck, 5–30 mm in diameter, diagnosed typically in adult life and more common in men than in women.

3.1.1.6 Eccrine poroma (Figs. 62, 63)

A nodular tumour of the acrosyringium.

Eccrine poromas are nodular tumours composed of lobules of squamoid cells, smaller than and sharply demarcated from the epithelium of the adjacent normal epidermis, with inconspicuous intercellular bridges and containing cytoplasmic glycogen. Most poromas contain small eccrine ducts. Some tumours include dermal components, whereas others are confined to the epidermis (*intra-epidermal epithelioma, hidroacanthoma simplex*). The overlying epidermis shows pronounced psoriasiform hyperplasia. Some tumours are composed entirely of lobular dermal components of identical pattern to the intra-epidermal tumours. This variant is known as *dermal duct tumour*.

Eccrine poromas occur most commonly on the palms and soles, but other areas including the head, neck and trunk may be involved.

3.1.1.7 Syringofibroadenoma (Fig. 64)

A fibroadenoma of eccrine ducts.

The tumour is composed of interconnecting slender cords of pale, cuboidal epithelium including small ductal structures, continuous with the hyperplastic epidermis. The strands of tumour cells enclose oedematous, vascular islands of stroma. Similar tumours with apocrine differentiation shown by decapitation secretion of columnar epithelium also occur.

These are rare, benign neoplasms usually occurring on the extremities of adults.

3.1.1.8 Nodular hidradenoma (eccrine acrospiroma, clear cell hidradenoma) (Fig. 65)

A lobulated, endophytic neoplasm of eccrine duct origin, either solid or cystic.

The tumour is usually circumscribed, although not encapsulated, commonly multilobular and solid or cystic. The solid component consists of polyhedral or fusiform cells with clear or eosinophilic cytoplasm. In those tumours which involve the epidermis, the superficial component resembles eccrine poroma. Cystic spaces containing sialomucin and ductal structures are often present, some lined by cuboidal epithelium, the others composed of concentric squamoid cells with only a small slit-like lumen.

Eccrine hidradenoma has no site predilection and usually presents as a solitary nodule, sometimes draining serous fluid.

3.1.1.9 Eccrine spiradenoma (Fig. 66)

A benign neoplasm combining elements of eccrine ductal and secretory epithelium.

Eccrine spiradenomas consist of one or several circumscribed nodules in the dermis or subcutis, composed of three types of cells. The largest cells have round or ovoid, pale nuclei and scant cytoplasm. Smaller cells with uniform, dark nuclei are admixed with the larger cells, forming aggregates and cords, and lymphocytes are often scattered throughout the nodule. The nodules are surrounded by a hyalinized basement membrane from which branching septa extend into the parenchyma, where small globules of the eosinophilic material are distributed throughout some segments of the tumour, presenting a pattern very similar to that of cylindroma.

Eccrine spiradenomas occur as solitary nodules or sometimes multiple, linear and zosteriform lesions. The tumours are painful and occur mainly on the trunk and extremities.

3.1.1.10 Cylindroma (Fig. 67)

A benign lobulated neoplasm composed of groups of epithelial cells surrounded by a prominent basement membrane.

The tumour consists of aggregates of two types of epithelium, larger cells with pale cytoplasm, mainly in the centres of cellular aggregates, and more peripheral, smaller cells with scant cytoplasm, mainly at the periphery of lobules along the thick basement membrane. Small ductal structures lined by cuboidal or flattened cuticular epithelium are present in most cylindromas. Globules of the hyalinized basement membrane material are also found between the epithelium in the tumour lobules. The presence of decapitation secretion in the ductal epithelium in rare cases has suggested apocrine differentiation.

Most cylindromas occur on the scalp as multiple nodules (turban tumour), more often in women. The origin of cylindroma is controversial, some authors believing that the lesion arises from apocrine glands, a theory that has not been confirmed by electron microscopy, whereas others have suggested that it originates in the eccrine duct.

3.1.2 Malignant

3.1.2.1 Sclerosing sweat duct carcinoma (syringomatous carcinoma, microcystic adnexal carcinoma) (Fig. 68)

A neoplasm of low-grade malignancy, composed of syringomatous structures arranged in an infiltrating growth pattern.

These tumours consist of small syringoid groups and cords of cuboidal or polyhedral cells, ductal structures and keratotic cysts in a fibrotic, sometimes densely sclerotic stroma. The proportions of cysts and ducts vary. The neoplastic cells are usually monomorphous, but more severe nuclear pleomorphism and numerous mitoses are seen in poorly differentiated tumours, which also show only focal, subtle duct formation. Invasion usually extends into the deep dermis or subcutis, frequently in association with perineural infiltration. Cytological atypia, an infiltrating growth pattern and perineural invasion distinguish this carcinoma from syringoma. In the superficial layers, the ductal structures may be very well differentiated, resembling syringoma or desmoplastic trichoepithelioma, especially when keratotic cysts are prominent, resulting in diagnostic difficulty or misdiagnosis when biopsies include only the superficial dermis. *Adenosquamous carcinoma*, characterized by pronounced squamous differentiation in the cells of the ductal structures, may represent a more aggressive variant of sclerosing sweat duct carcinoma.

Sclerosing sweat duct carcinomas occur most commonly in adults on the head and neck, mainly on the face, but also on the trunk and limbs. The neoplasms usually present as poorly defined zones of induration, enlarging slowly over a period of years with a tendency to recur.

3.1.2.2 Malignant mixed tumour of the skin (malignant chondroid syringoma) (Fig. 69)

A malignant version of benign mixed tumour of the skin (chondroid syringoma), including epithelial and prominent mesenchymal components.

These tumours are composed of lobular aggregates of polyhedral epithelial cells with eosinophilic or clear cytoplasm arranged in solid sheets and forming duct-like syringoid structures and keratotic cysts. The stroma includes cellular or hyalinized collagenous areas and myxoid or chondroid foci. Cytological atypia is present, although it is only slight in some cases, with nuclear atypia and few to numerous mitoses. An infiltrating growth pattern may be present. Loss of cohesion between tumour cells and a high proportion of chondroid or myxoid stroma containing single neoplastic cells or small aggregates are also indicators of malignancy.

These rare neoplasms present as slowly growing, smooth, nodular tumours, usually on the extremities.

3.1.2.3 Porocarcinoma (Fig. 70)

An eccrine carcinoma that may arise de novo or develop in established eccrine poroma as an entirely intra-epidermal tumour or with an invasive dermal component.

Porocarcinoma confined to the epidermis (in situ porocarcinoma) consists of circumscribed aggregates of small basaloid cells intermingled with larger, more atypical cells with pleomorphic nuclei and abnormal mitoses. The tumour may consist of small nests or more diffuse infiltration of the epidermis by single cells mimicking extramammary Paget disease. Tumours infiltrating the dermis are composed of islands of the smaller basaloid cells, possibly residual poroma, adjacent to sheets of much larger, atypical cells. Duct formation is usually present within the dermal nodules, including well-developed tubular structures lined by cuticular epithelium and poorly formed intracellular vacuoles.

Porocarcinoma occurs usually in elderly patients as verrucous or polypoid tumours on the head and neck or extremities.

3.1.2.4 Malignant nodular hidradenoma (Fig. 71)

A lobulated, deeply invasive adnexal neoplasm showing eccrine ductal and secretory differentiation, including a component of clear cells.

As with other malignant sweat gland carcinomas that have benign counterparts, these tumours, in contrast to the benign lesions, demonstrate irregular nodular architecture, infiltrative growth, increased mitotic activity, greater nuclear pleomorphism and, occasionally, vascular and lymphatic invasion.

This is a rare tumour, occurring mainly in elderly patients on the head and neck or extremities. Metastases are common.

3.1.2.5 Malignant eccrine spiradenoma (Fig. 72)

A malignant neoplasm apparently arising within a benign eccrine spiradenoma.

Severe cytological atypia and stromal infiltration distinguish these tumours from their benign counterparts.

The tumour is characterized clinically by rapid enlargement of a pre-existing nodule of the trunk or extremities.

3.1.2.6 Mucinous eccrine carcinoma (Fig. 73)

A nodular eccrine carcinoma characterized by atypical epithelial cells suspended in pools of mucin in the dermis.

Small groups, cords and single cuboidal epithelial cells with variable atypia and mitotic activity are suspended in pale basophilic sialomucin, divided into lobules by slender fibrous septa. Duct formation and cribriform patterns may be present.

These rare neoplasms occur most often on the head and neck, frequently on the eyelids of elderly patients. The tumours are slow growing and occasionally metastasize to regional lymph nodes, but rarely produce systemic metastases.

3.1.2.7 Adenoid cystic eccrine carcinoma (Fig. 74)

An eccrine neoplasm similar to adenoid cystic carcinoma of the salivary gland.

The tumour includes syringoid, ductal structures lined by cuboidal epithelium, solid groups of basaloid cells, cribriform and cystic structures, embedded in a fibrotic or mucinous stroma. Perineural invasion is usually present.

These rare tumours sometimes recur locally, but metastasis is rare.

3.1.2.8 Aggressive digital papillary adenoma/adenocarcinoma (Fig. 75)

A nodular or infiltrating eccrine neoplasm of the fingers, toes, palms and soles.

Poorly circumscribed nodular collections of ductal and alveolar structures contain papillary and cribriform areas. Malignant variants show more pronounced cytological atypia with poor glandular differentiation, focal necrosis and an infiltrating growth pattern.

These tumours have a high rate of local recurrence, and the adenocarcinomatous variant has a high metastatic rate.

3.2 Apocrine tumours

3.2.1 Benign

3.2.1.1 Apocrine cystadenoma (hidrocystoma) (Fig. 76)

A simple cystic benign neoplasm of apocrine glands.

The neoplasm is usually composed of a single cystic structure with a lining of one or several layers of cuboidal and columnar apocrine cells with eosinophilic cytoplasm and focal decapitation secretion. A layer of myoepithelial cells surrounds the epithelium. Small tufted collections of epithelial cells may project into the lumen, but true papillae are not present.

These tumours are usually solitary blue–black nodules of the head, neck or upper trunk.

3.2.1.2 Hidradenoma papilliferum (Fig. 77)

A benign apocrine neoplasm composed of cystic and papillary structures with a characteristic lace-like pattern.

The tumour is a circumscribed nodule in the dermis, usually separate from the epidermis and including cystic areas lined by flattened squamoid epithelium in the superficial segments and by an inner layer of tumour cells overlying peripheral cuboidal epithelium in the deep segments of the tumour. Papillary projections, often with a trabecular pattern, protrude into the lumina of the cystic areas. Decapitation secretion may be present in segments of the columnar epithelium. Plasma cells are not a feature.

These tumours usually occur as solitary nodules of the vulva and perianal regions of middle-aged women and less often on the eyelid, the nipple and in the external auditory canal.

3.2.1.3 Syringocystadenoma papilliferum (Fig. 78)

A benign cystic papillary neoplasm with apocrine ductal and secretory features and a stroma containing numerous plasma cells.

Papillary epidermal projections alternate with invaginations lined by squamous epithelium, leading into duct-like and cystic structures lined by an inner layer of columnar epithelium and a basal layer of cuboidal cells. The columnar cells have eosinophilic cytoplasm and basal nuclei and show decapitation secretion. A prominent feature is a dense infiltrate of plasma cells in the stroma.

These neoplasms arise as solitary, nodular or verrucous lesions, most commonly on the face or scalp. The tumours may be present at birth or develop in early childhood, frequently in association with naevus sebaceus.

3.2.1.4 Apocrine adenoma

A histologically diverse, benign apocrine neoplasm.

Apocrine adenoma may be predominantly solid, glandular, fibroadenomatous or tubular. The glandular structures are lined by a single layer of cells with eosinophilic cytoplasm and decapitation secretion. The apocrine fibroadenomas consist of ductal structures compressed by cellular fibrous stroma, resembling intracanalicular fibroadenoma of the breast. The tubular variant is composed of lobules of tubular structures lined by an inner layer of columnar cells with decapitation secretion, often with an outer layer of cuboidal cells and with small papillary projections into the lumina of the tubules.

Apocrine adenomas are usually solitary nodules of perianal or axillary skin and, less often, at other sites including the external auditory canal in association with ceruminous glands. The tubular variant sometimes occurs in association with naevus sebaceus.

3.2.1.5 Cylindroma (see 3.1.1.10)

3.2.2 Malignant

3.2.2.1 Apocrine adenocarcinoma (Fig. 79)

A cutaneous adenocarcinoma with apocrine differentiation and variable growth pattern.

The growth patterns may include solid, cystic, complex glandular, cribiform or tubular areas. The tumour cells have granular eosinophilic cytoplasm and may show decapitation secretion. Varied cytological atypia, mitotic activity and necrosis may be present. In some cases, normal apocrine gland lobules are present adjacent to the carcinoma with zones of transition between the benign and malignant apocrine epithelium.

These rare neoplasms occur most often in the axilla or anogenital regions.

3.3 Sebaceous gland tumours

3.3.1 Benign

3.3.1.1 Sebaceous adenoma (Fig. 80)

3.3.1.2 Sebaceous epithelioma (Fig. 81)

Benign neoplasms composed of multiple, circumscribed sebaceous gland lobules.

The tumour consists of multiple lobules connected to the epidermis which may be partially replaced by basaloid cells showing sebaceous differentiation. The lobules in the dermis consist of central collections of mature sebaceous cells, with peripheral layers of basaloid cells. In sebaceous adenoma the mature sebaceous cells form the majority of the cell population, whereas in sebaceous epithelioma the basaloid cells predominate.

Sebaceous adenoma and epithelioma are uncommon nodular tumours of the head and neck of older individuals.

3.3.2 Malignant

3.3.2.1 Sebaceous carcinoma (Fig. 82)

A highly malignant carcinoma showing sebaceous differentiation.

The tumour consists of irregular lobules, small groups and strands of atypical epithelium, including squamoid and basaloid cells as well as cells showing variable sebaceous differentiation with vacuolated cytoplasm containing lipid. Necrosis, nuclear pleomorphism and plentiful mitoses may be present.

Most sebaceous carcinomas occur on the eyelid in association with the glands of Zeiss and the meibomian glands. Extra-ocular sebaceous carcinoma is rare, occurring mainly on the head and neck of elderly patients as yellowish-pink or tan nodules. Sebaceous carcinomas may be associated with Muir-Torre syndrome.

3.3.3 Pilosebaceous hyperplasia and hamartomas

3.3.3.1 Follicular naevi

Hamartomatous malformations of the hair follicle. *The commonest forms are Becker pigmented hairy naevus, naevus comedonicus, hair follicle naevus and basaloid follicular hamartoma.*

Becker naevus. This lesion is characterized by an increase in the number of hair follicles, often associated with a hamartoma of arrector pili muscles, elongated rete ridges and hyperpigmentation of the basal layer.

Naevus comedonicus *(Fig. 83)*. A collection of dilated follicular infundibula plugged with keratin.

Hair follicle naevus. This lesion consists of a collection of small vellus hair follicles in a fibrovascular stroma.

Basaloid follicular hamartoma. Consists of cords and groups of basaloid cells, some of which are continuous with the walls of hair follicles, in a fibrotic stroma. Small keratin cysts may also be present.

Follicular naevi may be congenital or appear later in life. Becker naevus forms a plaque on the shoulder or chest, usually showing hyperpigmentation and hypertrichosis. Naevus comedonicus occurs as pigmented keratotic follicular plugs forming linear plaques. The hair follicle naevus presents as a small, smooth nodule or polypoid lesion. Basaloid follicular hamartoma presents as hyper- or hypopigmented indurated, linear plaques, often associated with hair loss.

3.3.3.2 Naevus sebaceus (Fig. 84)

A congenital hamartoma involving the epidermis, pilosebaceous complexes and other adnexal structures.

Early in life, the pilosebaceous complexes are immature, but sebaceous hyperplasia develops by puberty. Numerous small lobules of sebaceous glands are present in the superficial dermis, some communicating directly with the epidermal surface. Immature, malformed hair follicles are present, and apocrine glands are found in the deep dermis. Cutaneous neoplasms that develop within naevus sebaceus include basal cell carcinoma, syringocystadenoma papilliferum, hidradenoma, leiomyoma, sebaceous adenoma and trichilemmoma.

Naevus sebaceus occurs on the head and neck as a flat or verrucous hairless plaque, becoming more prominent and verrucous with age. A verrucous variant without a sebaceous component is termed naevus verrucosus.

3.3.3.3 Sebaceous gland hyperplasia

A localized abnormal increase in the number of sebaceous gland lobules grouped around a central hair follicle.

This lesion presents as small, yellowish papules on the face, particularly the forehead, of elderly persons.

3.4 Hair follicle tumours

3.4.1 Benign

3.4.1.1 Conical infundibular acanthoma (dilated pore) (Fig. 85)

A benign neoplasm of follicular infundibular epithelium.

The tumour consists of a dilated hair follicle plugged with keratin; proliferation of outer root sheath epithelium forms blunt projections into the adjacent stroma.

These lesions occur mainly on the head and neck of adults as small nodules with central comedones.

3.4.1.2 Pilar sheath acanthoma (Fig. 86)

A benign follicular infundibular tumour composed of epithelial lobules arising from the wall of a central cystic lesion.

Lobular outgrowths of outer root sheath epithelium protrude from the wall of a central cystically dilated hair follicle containing keratin, opening onto the epidermal surface through a pore-like ostium. The cells of the outer layers of the wall contain glycogen, and the central keratinization occurs via a granular layer.

Pilar sheath acanthoma occurs as a small nodule, usually on the upper lip.

3.4.1.3 Trichilemmoma (Fig. 87)

A benign neoplasm of hair follicles showing follicular infundibular and outer sheath differentiation.

The tumour is composed of one or more circumscribed lobules of glycogenated, squamoid epithelium usually continuous with the epidermis or follicular epithelium. A peripheral layer of palisaded basaloid cells overlies a thick hyalinized basement membrane. Small squamoid eddies and foci of keratinization may be present in the centre of the tumour.

Solitary trichilemmoma occurs as a small warty or smooth nodule on the skin of the face. Multiple trichilemmomas are manifestations of Cowden syndrome.

3.4.1.4 Tumour of follicular infundibulum (Fig. 88)

A benign tumour of follicular infundibulum resembling superficial basal cell carcinoma.

The tumour consists of a fenestrated, plate-like proliferation of glycogenated squamous epithelium in the superficial dermis with peripheral palisading of basal cells, connected to the epidermis by slender bridges of cells.

These lesions typically are solitary nodules of the head and neck.

3.4.1.5 Trichoepithelioma (epithelioma adenoides cysticum, superficial trichoblastoma) (Fig. 89)

A benign neoplasm of follicular germinative cells showing limited follicular differentiation.

The tumour is composed of lobular aggregates and cribriform strands of basaloid cells, surrounded by cellular, fibrous stroma. Peripheral palisading, foci of squamoid and sebaceous cells, and structures resembling hair bulbs and papillae may be present. Small keratinous cysts are present within the epithelial lobules, with focal calcification and pigmentation. Trichoepithelioma with abundant keratin cysts was previously termed *epithelioma adenoides cysticum*; those lesions including primitive hair bulbs and papillae are also known as *trichoblastoma* (Fig. 90).

Neoplasms of this type in which keratinous cysts predominate, with relatively little basaloid epithelial component, have been termed *trichoadenoma* (Fig. 91).

Desmoplastic trichoepithelioma (Fig. 92) refers to a variant in which small strands and lobules of basaloid epithelium are embedded in a dense sclerotic stroma with small keratinous cysts and focal calcification. The cell type and growth pattern are syringoid, indicating that this lesion may be a variant of syringoma.

Trichoepithelioma occurs as solitary (non-hereditary) and multiple (autosomal dominant) forms. Solitary lesions are pale, nodular tumours up to 2 cm in diameter, usually on the face of adults. Multiple trichoepitheliomas are small nodules of the face, scalp, neck and trunk in childhood which occur in association with cylindromas, syringomas and basal cell carcinoma.

3.4.1.6 Trichofolliculoma (Fig. 93)

A highly differentiated tumour of trichogenic epithelium including all elements of the pilosebaceous complex.

A central dilated hair follicle infundibulum contains keratin and multiple fine hair shafts, communicating with the epidermal surface through a dilated ostium. Numerous vellus follicles are attached to the wall of the central infundibulum and are surrounded by a sheath of cellular fibrous tissue. Sebaceous lobules may also be present in the secondary follicles.

Trichofolliculoma occurs typically as a solitary nodule of the face, scalp or neck. Fine white hairs usually emerge from a central pore. This lesion is probably a hamartoma or hair follicle naevus rather than a true neoplasm.

3.4.1.7 Pilomatricoma (Fig. 94)

A benign nodular neoplasm showing hair matrix and infundibular differentiation.

These tumours are situated in the deep dermis or subcutis and consist of nodular and cystic structures composed of sheets of basaloid cells merging with shadow (ghost) cells which have eosinophilic cytoplasm and pale or clear nuclear remnants. Aggregates of epithelium are embedded in cellular fibrous stroma containing histiocytes and foreign body type giant cells. Calcification and ossification may occur in aggregates of eosinophilic epithelial cells, but many tumours contain no calcification. In older lesions, only small aggregates of shadow cells remain, surrounded by fibrosis and giant cells with extensive calcification and only sparse basaloid epithelium.

Pilomatricoma is usually a solitary lesion, mainly of the face or upper extremity, occurring at any age, but frequently in children.

3.4.1.8 Pilar tumour (proliferating trichilemmal cyst) (Fig. 95)

A benign neoplasm representing the terminal stage in the growth of a proliferating trichilemmal cyst.

These tumours occur in the dermis or subcutis as circumscribed nodular lesions, sometimes with a peripheral layer of basaloid cells but composed mainly of large squamoid cells with abundant pale eosinophilic cytoplasm merging with compact orthokeratosis, without an intervening granular layer. Focal necrosis, mitotic activity and calcification may be present. Within the tumour there are numerous protruding aggregates of the pale squamoid epithelium and cystic collections of keratin.

This neoplasm usually occurs as a solitary nodular lesion on the scalp of elderly patients, more commonly in women.

3.4.2 Malignant

3.4.2.1 Trichilemmocarcinoma (Fig. 96)

The malignant counterpart of trichilemmoma.

The tumour is composed of lobules of large epithelial cells with clear or pale eosinophilic cytoplasm, atypical nuclei, mitoses and focal peripheral palisading. Abrupt keratinization of the trichilemmal type without a granular layer is present. The neoplastic lobules are attached to pilosebaceous units or to interfollicular epidermis, in which the neoplastic cells are sharply demarcated from normal epithelium.

Trichilemmocarcinoma is a raised, sometimes polypoid tumour of sun-exposed skin in elderly patients.

3.4.2.2 Malignant pilomatricoma (matrical carcinoma)

The malignant counterpart of pilomatricoma.

Malignant pilomatricoma is a nodular tumour of the dermis, sometimes involving the epidermis and extending into subcutaneous fat. Although composed, like its benign counterpart, of basaloid cells and shadow cells with fibrotic and granulomatous stroma, this neoplasm also demonstrates plentiful mitoses, focal necrosis and peripheral stromal infiltration by strands of atypical epithelium.

Malignant pilomatricoma is typically a solitary nodular tumour of the face, often greater than 1 cm in diameter. Most tumours are only locally invasive, and metastasis is rare.

3.4.3 Follicular cysts

3.4.3.1 Infundibular cyst (Fig. 97)

A cystic nodule of the dermis lined by stratified squamous epithelium with a granular layer surrounding laminated keratin.

The cysts may be small, involving vellus follicles (primary milia). Larger infundibular cysts may extend into the subcutis. The cyst wall resembles the epidermis or follicular infundibulum with a prominent granular layer, surrounding laminated keratin. The epithelial wall is frequently disrupted and replaced by histiocytes and giant cells in foci of rupture. The cyst may communicate with the epidermal surface through an ostium.

Infundibular cysts present as solitary or multiple smooth nodules on any cutaneous surface, but most often on the head, neck and trunk.

3.4.3.2 Trichilemmal cyst (pilar cyst) (Fig. 98)

A nodular cystic lesion derived from the isthmus of the hair follicle.

The wall is composed of an outer layer of basaloid cells surmounted by several layers of pale, eosinophilic squamous cells without a granular layer, surrounding compact, homogeneous keratin.

Trichilemmal cysts occur as smooth nodular lesions, single or multiple, mainly on the scalp.

3.4.3.3 Steatocystoma multiplex (Fig. 99)

A lesion composed of multiple dermal cysts showing pilosebaceous differentiation.

The cysts have thin, undulating walls of stratified squamous epithelium without a granular layer. Sebaceous lobules are present in the wall or in the adjacent stroma; one pilar unit is associated with each cyst, which may contain lanugo hairs.

Multiple cysts occur in presternal skin, the proximal extremities, face, scalp and axillae. They may be sporadic or familial with autosomal dominant inheritance.

3.4.3.4 Dermoid cyst (Fig. 100)

A rare subcutaneous cyst lined by squamous epithelium with skin appendages in the wall.

The wall is composed of stratified squamous epithelium with a granular layer, similar to that of an infundibular cyst. Hair follicles radiate from the cyst wall into the adjacent stroma, and sebaceous glands, eccrine glands and occasionally apocrine glands may also be present in the stroma.

Dermoid cysts are found typically at or soon after birth along lines of embryonic fusion, most often on the head and neck and particularly adjacent to the outer canthus of the eye.

3.4.3.5 Eruptive vellus hair cyst (Fig. 101)

A small dermal cyst containing vellus hairs in a dilated follicular infundibulum.

The cyst is lined by stratified squamous epithelium with focal trichilemmal keratinization. Segments of vellus hair shafts and keratin are present in the lumen. Some cysts are connected to the epidermis through a small ostium, and in some cases a telogen follicle is contiguous with the inferior segment of the cyst.

Multiple small papules occur mainly on the chest and axillae of children and young adults.

3.4.4 Tumours of pilosebaceous mesenchyme

3.4.4.1 Follicular fibroma (trichodiscoma, fibrofolliculoma, perifollicular fibroma)

Three distinct types of benign proliferations of perifollicular mesenchyme recapitulating the hair disc, fibrous sheath or papilla.

Trichodiscoma. This is a sharply defined fibrovascular lesion of the superficial dermis, sometimes occurring in association with a hair follicle. The overlying epidermis is flattened, and connective tissue mucin is present between the loose fascicles of fibrous tissue in the tumour.

Fibrofolliculoma. This lesion consists of proliferation of perifollicular stroma, with compact collagen and fibroblasts surrounding one or more distorted hair follicles from which interlocking strands of basaloid cells push into the surrounding fibrous tissue.

Perifollicular fibroma (Fig. 102). This lesion consists of perifollicular proliferation of cellular fibrous tissue without the interlocking strands of proliferating epithelium as seen in fibrofolliculoma.

These lesions occur as multiple papules, usually on the face. Multiple fibrofolliculomas and trichodiscomas may occur in association with fibro-epithelial polyps.

4 Paget Disease

4.1 Mammary Paget disease

4.2 Extramammary Paget disease (Fig. 103)

An intra-epidermal proliferation of atypical mucin-producing epithelial cells, with or without an underlying carcinoma of adnexal or visceral origin.

The epidermis, which is usually hyperplastic, contains atypical epithelial cells with clear or pale cytoplasm distributed singly or in groups at all levels of the epidermis. The nuclei are large, with prominent nucleoli; mitoses are usually present. The cells frequently extend into the walls of hair follicles and eccrine ducts. In most cases with dermal invasion there is an associated adnexal carcinoma or carcinoma of underlying organs including rectum, prostate, bladder, cervix and urethra.

Most cases occur in the skin of the vulva, male genitalia, groin or perianal region. The origin of extramammary Paget disease is controversial. A large proportion of cases is not associated with underlying adenocarcinoma; in these cases, the intra-epidermal carcinoma is thought to arise from apocrine progenitor cells or other pluripotent cells in the epidermis.

---

[1] See WHO (1981) Histological typing of breast tumours, International Histological Classification of Tumours, 2nd edn. World Health Organization, Geneva.

5 Cutaneous Lymphoproliferative Tumours

5.1 Cutaneous T-cell lymphoma

A primary T-cell lymphoma of the skin.

5.1.1 Mycosis fungoides
(Fig. 104)

Mycosis fungoides in most cases first becomes evident in the patch stage, followed by evolution into plaque and tumour or nodule stages. In some cases, however, the plaque stage appears to develop de novo. Involvement of all cutaneous surfaces may be very extensive in the plaque and tumour stages. Erythroderma may occur during any of the three stages of mycosis fungoides.

Patch stage. The epidermis characteristically shows psoriasiform hyperplasia overlying a perivascular and diffuse lymphocytic infiltrate, sometimes relatively sparse, in the superficial dermis. The lymphocytes may be closely applied to the basal layer of the epidermis in a focally lichenoid pattern; fibrosis is present in the superficial stroma, where coarse bundles of collagen replace the normal delicate fibrils of the papillary dermis. Epidermotropism of atypical lymphocytes with hyperchromatic, irregular (cerebriform) nuclei is an important feature. These cells may be arranged singly or in small collections between the keratinocytes, sometimes associated with slight spongiosis, but only rarely with spongiotic vesicles. There is also a poikilodermatous form of patch-stage mycosis fungoides in which the epidermis is atrophic, with alternating hyper- and hypopigmentation and telangiectasia in the superficial dermis. Epidermotropism may be subtle in the patch stage, an early sign being the presence of lymphocytes in a beaded pattern between the epithelial cells of the basal layer.

Plaque stage. In the plaque stage there is a denser infiltrate of lymphocytes in the papillary and superficial reticular dermis, composed of atypical lymphoid cells with hyperchromatic nuclei, markedly convoluted nuclear membranes (cerebriform nuclei), plasma cells, larger cells with pale cytoplasm, vesicular nuclei and prominent nucleoli resembling Reed-Sternberg cells, and eosinophils. Epidermotropism is more pronounced with formation of collections of atypical lymphoid cells (Pautrier microabscesses). Lymphocytic infiltration of the epithelium of adnexal structures is often present, sometimes with associated excessive mucin deposition in and degeneration of follicles (follicular mucinosis).

Tumour stage. In this stage there is a deep and dense dermal infiltrate composed of sheets of lymphoid cells with infiltration of adnexal structures. The cell population is more monomorphous, composed predominantly of atypical, pleomorphic lymphoid cells including large immunoblast-like cells. Epidermotropism is absent or sparse, and the papillary dermis also is often spared.

Variants

Spongiotic mycosis fungoides. In some cases spongiosis with vesicle formation may co-exist with epidermotropism of atypical lymphoid cells in non-spongiotic areas.

Hypereosinophilic mycosis fungoides. Although eosinophils are frequently present, especially in the plaque stage of mycosis fungoides, in some cases they are much more plentiful, forming dense groups and sheets, outnumbering the lymphoid cells in some areas.

Granulomatous mycosis fungoides. Some cases of mycosis fungoides are characterized by a prominent granulomatous component in the infiltrate, composed of epithelioid histiocytes in a diffuse or more localized pattern, resembling sarcoidosis or tuberculoid leprosy.

Granulomatous slack skin (Fig. 105)**.** This rare condition may be a variant of granulomatous mycosis fungoides in which there is extensive elastophagocytosis by macrophages and giant cells leading to the formation of loose folds of skin, especially in the groin and axillae.

5.1.2 Sezary syndrome

Cutaneous T-cell lymphoma in association with circulating neoplastic T-lymphocytes in the peripheral blood.

5.1.3 Pagetoid reticulosis (Woringer-Kollop disease)

A type of cutaneous T-cell lymphoma characterized by an infiltrate of atypical T-lymphocytes localized to the epidermis.

The epidermis is hyperplastic and infiltrated by lymphocytes with large, hyperchromatic, convoluted nuclei arranged either singly or in Pautrier microabscess-like collections in lacunae. The underlying dermis contains only small lymphocytes. The epithelium of adnexal structures is frequently involved by the atypical lymphocytic infiltrate. The neoplastic cells are T-lymphocytes, probably of the suppressor type, unlike those of classical mycosis fungoides, which are of the helper type.

Pagetoid reticulosis is typically a solitary hyperkeratotic plaque on the hands or feet, occurring almost exclusively in men, most commonly in the sixth and seventh decades of life. Progression to disseminated lesions or systemic disease is rare; in most cases the disease pursues a benign course.

5.1.4 Adult T-cell leukaemia/lymphoma

A clinical variant of cutaneous T-cell lymphoma resulting from human T-cell leukaemia virus (HTLV)-1 retrovirus infection.

The dermis is infiltrated by atypical, pleomorphic T-lymphocytes, similar to the infiltrate of non-epidermotropic (tumour stage) mycosis fungoides.

These patients present with the rapid onset of papules, plaques and nodules on the trunk and extremities, sometimes associated with erythroderma. The cutaneous lesions are always associated with visceral involvement.

5.2 Cutaneous B-cell lymphoma (Fig. 106)

A primary B-cell lymphoma of the skin.

Precise classification of B-cell lymphoma is usually not possible on the basis of the skin biopsy appearances alone, but the following types may be represented:

1. Small B-lymphocytic
2. Plasmacytoid lymphocytic
3. Immunoblastic sarcoma of B-cells
4. Lymphomas of follicular centre cells
   a) Small cleaved cell
   b) Large cleaved cell

c) Small non-cleaved cell
d) Large non-cleaved cell
5. Lymphoblastic lymphoma (rare B-cell subtypes)

Cutaneous B cell lymphoma, whether arising primarily in the skin or in systemic lymphoma, infiltrates the dermis in a diffuse or nodular pattern, sparing the papillary dermis and epidermis. The infiltrate is frequently densest in the deeper layers, in contrast to most benign lymphocytic infiltrates. The lymphoid cells form nodular aggregates around vessels and adnexal structures or diffuse sheets of cells which may extend into the subcutis. The infiltrate is composed of monomorphous neoplastic lymphocytes showing the cytological characteristics of their primary nodal lymphoma counterpart. In primary *cutaneous follicular lymphoma* (Fig. 107), differentiation from cutaneous follicular hyperplasia may be extremely difficult. Helpful distinguishing features of lymphoma include the following: absence of tingible body macrophages, thin or absent follicular mantles, a monomorphic population within follicles (with the exception of follicular mixed lymphoma) and low mitotic rate in follicles.

Malignant angioendotheliomatosis (Fig. 108) is a form of B-cell lymphoma characterized by dilated blood vessels containing atypical lymphoid cells adherent to the endothelial surface.

Primary cutaneous involvement by B-cell lymphoma occurs in only a small proportion of patients. Cutaneous involvement in patients with nodal B-cell lymphoma is found in less than 5% of patients. The cutaneous nodules may be single or multiple, occurring most often on the head, neck and trunk.

5.3 Cutaneous plasmacytoma

Primary or secondary cutaneous infiltration of benign or malignant B lymphocytes with terminal differentiation features of plasma cells.

The pattern of dermal infiltration may be diffuse or nodular, sparing the papillary dermis and epidermis. The neoplastic cells range from well-differentiated plasmacytoid cells to highly atypical forms with pleomorphic, hyperchromatic nuclei, plentiful mitoses and binucleated cells.

Primary malignant cutaneous plasmacytomas are rare. Secondary malignant cutaneous plasmacytomas are the metastatic lesions of multiple myeloma or plasma cell leukaemia. The lesions appear as single or multiple plaques and nodules of red to purplish colour without epidermal scaling or ulceration.

5.4 Cutaneous lymphoma, pleomorphic variants

5.4.1 T-immunoblastic lymphoma

Lesions of mycosis fungoides and Sezary syndrome in which transformation into immunoblastic lymphoma has taken place.

Dense nodular or diffuse infiltrates extend through the full thickness of the dermis into the subcutis. The lymphoid cells are large with ovoid vesicular nuclei, large nucleoli and basophilic or pale cytoplasm. Mitoses are plentiful, and the infiltrate includes numerous histiocytes.

T-immunoblastic lymphoma occurs as solitary or multiple cutaneous nodules.

5.4.2 Large cell anaplastic lymphoma (Fig. 109)

A lymphoma composed of very large, pleomorphic lymphoid cells resembling histiocytes or Reed-Sternberg cells.

A dense infiltrate of lymphoid cells extends through the dermis into the subcutis without epidermotropism. The cells are large with round or pleomorphic nuclei, prominent nucleoli and abundant pale cytoplasm. The infiltrate often includes giant cells resembling Reed-Sternberg cells. Most tumour cells express the activation antigen CD30 (Ki-1), as do the large atypical cells of Hodgkin lymphoma, some advanced cases of mycosis fungoides, lymphomatoid papulosis and regressing atypical histiocytosis.

The clinical lesions are rapidly growing, reddish or violaceous cutaneous plaques and nodules.

5.5 Dysplastic lymphocytic proliferations (lymphomatoid vasculitis)

A group of disorders characterized by cutaneous infiltration by dysplastic lymphocytes, vascular damage and a variable tendency for evolution into lymphoma. This group includes lymphomatoid papulosis, lymphomatoid granulomatosis and angioimmuno-blastic lymphadenopathy.

5.5.1 **Lymphomatoid papulosis** (Fig. 110)

A T cell lymphoproliferative disorder appearing in crops of papular lesions, most of which regress spontaneously.

Lymphomatoid papulosis shows a dense, wedge-shaped dermal infiltrate of atypical lymphoid cells, small lymphocytes, eosinophils and neutrophils. The blood vessels are often thick-walled with prominent endothelium. Lymphomatoid papulosis comprises two types based on the morphology of the atypical lymphoid cells. In type A lymphomatoid papulosis (histiocytic type), the atypical cells are large mononuclear cells with pale nuclei and prominent nucleoli resembling Reed-Sternberg cells. In type B lymphomatoid papulosis (lymphocytic type), the predominant cells are lymphoid cells with cerebriform nuclei.

The lesions appear mainly on the trunk and limbs of women in the third and fourth decades of life. Although most lesions regress spontaneously, progression to systemic lymphoma has been documented in approximately 10% of patients.

5.5.2 **Lymphomatoid granulomatosis** (Fig. 111)

A form of pulmonary vasculitis and granulomatosis which frequently has extrapulmonary manifestations.

This condition is a dermal infiltrate, densest in the deep dermis (bottom heavy), composed of angiocentric and angiodestructive nodules of large lymphoid cells with cleaved nuclei, predominantly T-cells. Lymphomatoid granulomatosis shares some features with angiocentric T-cell lymphoma, to which it is closely related.

The cutaneous lesions are erythematous papules, plaques and nodules, often ulcerated. Pulmonary involvement always occurs, but cutaneous lesions, seen in up to 60% of cases, may sometimes develop before the pulmonary manifestation.

5.5.3 **Angioimmunoblastic lymphadenopathy (with dysproteinaemia)**

A systemic disorder characterized by generalized lymphadenopathy, hepatosplenomegaly, fever, anaemia and polyclonal gammopathy with cutaneous involvement in approximately one third of cases.

The dermal infiltrate in this condition is polymorphous, containing plasmacytoid cells and immunoblasts in perivascular distribution in the superficial and deep dermis.

The cutaneous involvement consists of maculopapular and nodular lesions.

5.6 Langerhans cell histiocytosis (histiocytosis X) (Fig. 112)

A proliferation of Langerhans cells occurring in several clinically distinctive forms with variably aggressive biological potential.

There is considerable overlap between the histological features of the variants of histiocytosis X. Infiltrates may be localized at the superficial dermis in a band-like distribution or arranged in nodular or diffuse patterns throughout the upper dermis. Epidermotropism is frequently present, and the hair follicles may also be involved. The atypical Langerhans cells have pale vesicular or denser eosinophilic cytoplasm, large pale nuclei with small nucleoli and indented or cleaved nuclear membranes presenting a reniform contour. Eosinophils are frequently present. The neoplastic Langerhans cells react positively for S100 protein in formalin-fixed tissue and for CD1 antigen in frozen tissue.

Letterer-Siwe disease is a rare and lethal variant, usually affecting young children below the age of 3 years, presenting maculopapular and erythematous skin lesions. Hand-Schuller-Christian disease is also rare, affecting young children and, less commonly, adults, producing the triad of exophthalmos, diabetes insipidus and cranial deposits. Maculopapular skin lesions occur on the chest, axillae and groin. Eosinophilic granuloma (Langerhans cell granuloma, localized histiocytosis X of the skin) is a benign disorder of older children and adults, often forming solitary lytic bone lesions but also involving extra-osseous sites including the skin and the mucosae. Crusted papules or nodules occur on the face, scalp and axillae.

5.7 Regressing atypical histiocytosis

A dermal lymphocytic infiltrate characterized by repeated regression and recurrence, developing in some cases into persistent disease, probably a form of cutaneous T cell lymphoma, although the histogenesis is controversial.

The lesion shows epidermal hyperplasia and frequently ulceration overlying a dense mononuclear cellular infiltrate in the dermis, including a preponderance of large atypical cells with amphophilic cytoplasm, pleomorphic nuclei and large nucleoli, resembling Reed-Sternberg cells. Mixed inflammatory cells, granulation tissue, fibrosis and eosinophils may be present in the intervening stroma. Exclusion of other lymphoproliferative entities leaves very few cases in this category.

Recurrent, rapidly developing, ulcerated nodules eventually develop into persistent lesions.

5.8 Mastocytosis (Fig. 113)

A spectrum of related diseases in which there is an increase in mast cells in one or more organs. Cutaneous mastocytosis occurs as urticaria pigmentosa, solitary mastocytoma, diffuse cutaneous mastocytosis and telangiectasia macularis eruptiva perstans (TMEP).

According to the clinical variant of the disease, there may be only a very slight increase in the number of superficial perivascular mast cells as in telangiectasia macularis eruptiva perstans, more obvious perivascular aggregates of mast cells in urticaria pigmentosa, a diffuse infiltrate in disseminated cutaneous mastocytosis, and dense aggregates of mast cells in solitary mastocytoma. The mast cells may be ovoid, round or fusiform, and their cytoplasm may show obvious granularity or be almost clear, depending on the degree of degranulation. Toluidine blue, Giemsa and chloroacetate esterase are useful in staining the metachromatic granules. The superficial dermis may be oedematous; eosinophils frequently accompany the mast cell infiltrate, and the basal layer of the epidermis may be hyperpigmented.

Urticaria pigmentosa is the most common variant, occurring most often in children as multiple maculopapular lesions. Solitary mastocytosis occurs as one or several pruritic nodules. The skin lesions of systemic mastocytosis are similar to those of urticaria pigmentosa. Telangiectasia macularis eruptiva perstans occurs in adults as erythematous, telangiectatic, pigmented macules.

5.9 Leukaemia cutis (Fig. 114)

Secondary dermal infiltration by malignant haemopoietic cells of acute or chronic myelogenous or lymphocytic leukaemia.

Leukaemic infiltration of the dermis occurs in a variety of patterns but may mimic benign dermatoses (perivascular pattern) or cutaneous lymphoma, mainly of the B lymphocyte type (nodular or diffuse patterns). Infiltration by chronic lymphocytic leukaemia is indistinguishable from small cell (well-differentiated) lymphocytic lymphoma. The blast cells of acute granulocytic leukaemias may be confused with those of large cell lymphoma, whereas the cells of chronic granulocytic leukaemia may represent a range of differentiation, including mature and immature myeloid cells.

Cutaneous leukaemic infiltration presents as pinkish-red, purpuric papules, nodules and indurated plaques. Infiltrates of granulocytic leukaemia present a greenish colour due to their content of myeloperoxidase (chloromas).

6 Vascular Tumours

6.1 Benign

6.1.1 Capillary haemangioma[1]

6.1.2 Cavernous haemangioma[1]

6.1.3 Angiokeratoma (Fig. 115)

A capillary haemangioma in the superficial dermis closely applied to the overlying hyperplastic epidermis.

The epidermis is raised, often with irregular acanthosis overlying dilated, thin-walled blood vessels, some of which appear to be surrounded by interlocking rete ridges. Organized thrombi are frequently present in the blood vessels.

Angiokeratomas occur as four clinical types: angiokeratoma of Mibelli occurring on the dorsa of the fingers and toes, angiokeratoma of Fordyce affecting the scrotal skin, solitary papular angiokeratoma and the diffuse systemic angiokeratoma corporis diffusum associated with Fabry disease. The lesions of Fabry disease are similar to other angiokeratomas, without the hyperkeratosis frequently associated with the other types. Lipid

---

[1] Defined as in Weiss SW (1994) Histological typing of soft tissue tumours, WHO International Histological Classification of Tumours. Springer-Verlag, Berlin Heidelberg New York.

deposition is present in the endothelial and muscle cells of small blood vessels in the skin.

6.1.4 Verrucous keratotic haemangioma

A capillary and cavernous haemangioma of the superficial and deep dermis associated with verruciform hyperplasia of the overlying epidermis.

These lesions simulate angiokeratoma in their superficial portions, but the vascular component extends also into the deep dermis and subcutis.

Verrucous keratotic haemangioma occurs mainly on the legs of children, enlarging with age to produce wart-like lesions.

6.1.5 Tufted haemangioma (Fig. 116)

A capillary haemangioma occurring as multiple red plaques of the skin on the upper trunk or neck of children.

The tumour is composed of circumscribed collections of thin-walled blood vessels in the dermis. Aggregates of plump spindle cells, probably pericytes, form bulging invaginations in a semi-lunar shape.

6.1.6 Spindle cell angioendothelioma

A spindle cell vascular neoplasm with the biological potential of a low-grade angiosarcoma.

The lesion consists of numerous, irregular, dilated blood vessels in the dermis and subcutis. Intraluminal thrombi are present within some vessels, and in the intervening stroma there is haemorrhage, with foci of spindle cell and epithelial cell proliferation.

Spindle cell angioendothelioma forms reddish nodular tumours of the distal extremities, mainly in boys and men below the age of 25.

6.1.7 Glomus tumour (Fig. 117)

6.1.8 Glomangioma (Fig. 118)

Benign neoplasms of dermal glomus cells, with accompanying angiomatous proliferation in the case of glomangioma.

Glomus tumours are composed of small vessels surrounded by solid aggregates of uniform glomus cells. Glomangiomas consist of collections of dilated vessels surrounded by a few layers of uniform glomus cells.

Solitary glomus tumours are small, painful nodules of the extremities, often located in the nail bed. Multiple glomus tumours and glomangiomas are of varied size, localized or diffuse and may be painful or without symptoms.

6.2 Malignant

6.2.1 Kaposi sarcoma (Fig. 119)

A vascular proliferation of unknown pathogenesis, possibly a reactive process rather than a true neoplasm. Four clinico-pathological types occur: the indolent classic type, the African (endemic) type, an aggressive systemic form associated with immunosuppressive therapy and Kaposi sarcoma associated with the acquired immunodeficiency syndrome (AIDS).

The histological features of the different clinical types of Kaposi sarcoma are the same. In patch-stage Kaposi sarcoma, the changes are subtle, consisting of a slight increase in the number of vessels in the superficial dermis lined by flattened or prominent endothelial cells. The vessels are thin walled, dilated and of irregular outline and may surround a pre-existing vessel (the promontory sign). Lymphocytes, plasma cells, erythrocytes and haemosiderin deposition are present in the intervening stroma, in which there may be an increase in the number of spindle cells surrounding slit-like spaces. In the more advanced plaques and nodules of Kaposi sarcoma, there are denser collections of spindle cells in the dermis forming sheets and nodular aggregates containing slit-like spaces with an associated inflammatory infiltrate of lymphocytes and plasma cells. The spindle cells may be uniform or show moderate nuclear pleomorphism and hyperchromatism, with mitotic figures in varied numbers. Extravasation of erythrocytes is prominent, and small, eosinophilic hyaline globules may be seen in the interstitium or within the cytoplasm of spindle cells and macrophages. These bodies probably represent phagocytosed fragments of erythrocytes.

The irregularity of the vessels, the banal morphology of the endothelium and the presence of plasma cells and eosinophilic globules are important features in distinguishing Kaposi sarcoma from other vascular proliferations such as acroangiodermatitis and from angiosarcoma. Current evidence suggests that the spindle cell component of Kaposi sarcoma shows endothelial differentiation, but it remains controversial as to whether these cells are of blood vessel or lymphatic endothelial origin.

Patients with Kaposi sarcoma in the patch stage present with small lesions similar to petechiae or ecchymoses. The lesions enlarge with time to form violaceous plaques and tumours which may ulcerate. The indolent classic Kaposi sarcoma usually affects elderly patients of Mediterranean or Askanazy Jewish origin, forming lesions mainly of the lower extremities which pursue a chronic, non-lethal course. The African type includes three main subtypes, most commonly a nodular form similar to classic Kaposi sarcoma with a benign course, a more aggressive subtype characterized by extensive skin lesions and a lymphadenopathic type occurring mainly in children. The more aggressive types associated with immunosuppressive therapy and AIDS are characterized by more extensive, more rapidly progressive lesions associated with a poor prognosis. The multiple lesions in these cases, however, may be a manifestation of multifocal distribution rather than true metastasis.

6.2.2 **Angiosarcoma** (Fig. 120)

A malignant neoplasm of blood vessel type (haemangiosarcoma, malignant haemangioendothelioma, haemangioblastoma).

These tumours demonstrate a range of microscopic appearances including obviously angiomatoid areas and more compact nodules and sheets of spindle or epithelioid cells surrounding inconspicuous slit-like spaces. Atypical vascular structures may form anastomosing networks or dissect between the collagen bundles of the dermal stroma, with infiltration into the subcutis. The endothelial cells show varied nuclear atypia and may form several layers or small bulging tufts. A lymphocytic infiltrate is frequently present in the interstitium, with dilated lymphatic vessels at the periphery of the tumour lobules. Mitoses may be plentiful in the more solid areas. Positive immunostaining for factor VIII and negative staining for S100 protein may be helpful in distinguishing poorly differentiated angiosarcoma from other spindle cell neoplasms. The presence of bulging, atypical endothelial cells and anastomosing vascular channels and the absence of cytoplasmic globules help to distinguish angiosarcoma from some nodular forms of Kaposi sarcoma.

Angiosarcoma occurs either de novo on the head and neck of elderly patients as single or multiple plaques and nodules that may ulcerate or in a lymphadenomatous extremity, usually in the upper arm following radical mastectomy (Stewart-Treves syndrome).

6.3 Vascular malformations

6.3.1 Naevus flammeus

6.3.2 Hereditary haemorrhagic telangiectasia

6.3.3 Angioma serpiginosum

Congenital or acquired vascular lesions characterized by telangiectasia.

The lesions of all congenital vascular malformations share the common feature of telangiectasia, with varying degrees of vascular proliferation and thickness of blood vessel walls.

Naevus flammeus presents as two clinical forms, the salmon patch which involutes and the persistent port wine stain. The port wine stain may be associated with Sturge-Weber syndrome and Klippel-Trenaunay-Weber syndrome. Hereditary haemorrhagic telangiectasia (Osler-Weber-Rendu disease) is characterized by multiple, small red papules on the skin and mucous membranes in childhood. Angioma serpiginosum occurs as pinhead-sized papules on the extremities of children, frequently arranged in arcuate or serpiginous patterns.

6.4 Vascular hyperplasias

Vascular hyperplasias composed of proliferations of endothelial cells accompanying inflammatory and reparative processes may be confused with true neoplasia, hence their inclusion in this volume.

6.4.1 Acroangiodermatitis

A vasoproliferative disorder associated with venous stasis.

Blood vessels with plump endothelial cells form small collections similar to those seen in stasis dermatitis in the superficial dermis. Fibroplasia, a sparse lymphocytic infiltrate and siderophages are present in the stroma.

Acroangiodermatitis occurs as violaceous papules and nodules of the lower legs and feet of patients with venous stasis, paralysis of a limb or congenital arteriovenous malformation. The lesions resemble Kaposi sarcoma clinically and histologically, hence the synonym "pseudo-Kaposi sarcoma".

6.4.2 Intravascular papillary endothelial hyperplasia

A form of organization of a thrombus within a vein or a vascular malformation, characterized by papillary protrusions of endothelium.

Papillary invaginations of endothelial cells protrude into a distorted vascular lumen in the deep dermis involving either a pre-existing haemangioma or vein. The presence of thrombosis in some cases indicates that the lesion is a form of organizing thrombus.

These small nodular lesions of the head, neck and hands most often affect middle-aged and older women.

6.4.3 Bacillary angiomatosis (Fig. 121)

A reactive tumour-like vascular proliferation associated with HIV infection.

The lesions resemble pyogenic granuloma and epithelioid haemangioma, consisting of lobular collections of small blood vessels, often with a collarette of epidermis. Protuberant endothelial cells show nuclear pleomorphism and numerous mitoses. Neutrophils and nuclear dust are present in the stroma, with clumps of granular basophilic material representing rickettsia-like bacilli that stain positively with the Warthin-Starry method.

This lesion occurs mainly, but not exclusively in AIDS patients and may be confused clinically and histologically with Kaposi sarcoma, from which it is distinguished by demonstration of the bacilli.

6.4.4 Pyogenic granuloma (lobular haemangioma, haemangioma of granulation tissue type) (Fig. 122)

A common benign vascular tumour of skin and mucous membranes characterized by lobular collections of capillaries producing a polypoid or sessile lesion. Pyogenic granuloma may be regarded as a true haemangioma or a reactive proliferation of granulation tissue.

The epidermis is raised, attenuated and frequently ulcerated overlying lobulated collections of capillaries in the dermis, often with oedema and a mixed inflammatory infiltrate. At the margins of the tumour, the epidermis frequently forms elongated rete ridges in a collarette pattern.

Pyogenic granuloma is usually a solitary red to brown or polypoid lesion of the face, fingers, lips or gingiva.

6.4.5 Angiolymphoid hyperplasia with eosinophilia (epithelioid haemangioma, histiocytoid haemangioma) (Fig. 123)

A violaceous, nodular, angiolymphoid proliferation occurring most often in auricular or peri-auricular skin.

The lesion is composed of lobular collections of small blood vessels lined by epithelioid endothelial cells with an infiltrate of lymphocytes and eosinophils in the intervening stroma.

These nodular lesions of auricular and peri-auricular skin are possibly related to arthropod bite and resolve spontaneously. Kimura disease, a similar angioproliferative process affecting young male patients of Oriental extraction, is probably a distinct disorder.

7 Lymphatic Tumours[1]

7.1 Benign

7.1.1 Capillary lymphangioma

7.1.2 Cavernous lymphangioma

7.1.3 Cystic lymphangioma (hygroma)

7.2 Malignant

7.2.1 Lymphangiosarcoma (malignant lymphangioendothelioma)

[1] See Weiss SW (1994) Histological typing of soft tissue tumours, WHO International Histological Classification of Tumours. Springer-Verlag, Berlin Heidelberg New York.

8 Cutaneous Fibrohistiocytic Tumours

8.1 Benign

8.1.1 Benign fibrous histiocytoma (dermatofibroma, histiocytoma, sclerosing haemangioma) (Fig. 124)

A benign neoplasm of dermal spindle cells, including histiocytes.

The epidermis is usually hyperplastic with hyperpigmentation of the basal layer, separated by a clear (grenz) zone from the spindle cell tumour in the dermis which includes fibroblast-like spindle cells, histiocytes and blood vessels in varying proportions. In some lesions the spindle cells may be distributed singly between the collagen bundles, forming a subtle zone of increased cellularity, whereas in larger tumours there is much denser cellularity, including spindle cells with elongated or ovoid, vesicular nuclei arranged in sheets or interlocking strands in storiform pattern, embedded in a loose collagenous stroma. Foamy histiocytes and giant cells may be present in large numbers in xanthomatous areas.

Variants

8.1.1.1 Cellular benign fibrous histiocytoma

A very densely cellular tumour with fascicular and storiform growth patterns and frequent extension into the subcutis. The neoplasm shares some features, therefore, with dermatofibrosarcoma protuberans, from which it is distinguished by the epidermal hyperplasia, its more polymorphic cell population, hyalinized collagen surrounded by tumour cells at the edge of the lesion and absence of immunostaining for CD34 (human haemopoietic progenitor cell antigen).

8.1.1.2 Aneurysmal benign fibrous histiocytoma

Collections of capillaries, foci of haemorrhage and siderophages and foamy macrophages surround cleft-like and cavernous blood-filled spaces in the centre of the tumour, which otherwise shows typical features of benign fibrous histiocytoma. Aneurysmal benign fibrous histiocytoma is distinguished from *angiomatoid fibrous histiocytoma* by the presence in the latter tumour of monomorphic histiocyte-like cells with a prominent lymphocytic infiltrate and its presentation in a younger age group, occasionally with systemic symptoms, usually in a subcutaneous location.

8.1.1.3 Epithelioid benign fibrous histiocytoma

A distinctive form characterized by epithelioid cells with abundant eosinophilic cytoplasm, binucleate cells, foamy macrophages and spindle cells forming a polypoid tumour with an epidermal collarette.

8.1.1.4 Atypical (pseudosarcomatous) benign fibrous histiocytoma

This tumour is characterized by a component of pleomorphic cells with hyperchromatic nuclei in addition to the spindle cells, foamy macrophages and giant cells of common benign fibrous histiocytoma.

These very common tumours are found on all cutaneous surfaces, but most commonly on the extremities. They are usually less than 10mm in diameter, firm and nodular, flat or depressed. Abundant histiocytes containing lipid and haemosiderin in some cases give the cut surface a yellowish to brown hue.

8.1.2 Dermatomyofibroma

A benign dermal plaque-like proliferation of fibroblasts and myofibroblasts.

Uniform spindle cells in elongated and intersecting fascicles mainly arranged parallel to the epidermal surface form a well-circumscribed plaque in the reticular dermis and may extend into the upper subcutis. Immunocytochemical reactivity for vimentin and non-specific muscle actin and the ultrastructural features suggest myofibroblastic differentiation in this recently described neoplasm.

Dermatomyofibroma occurs mainly in young adults, more commonly in women and most frequently in the shoulder region.

8.1.3 Benign (juvenile) xanthogranuloma (Fig. 125)

A nodular infiltrate of non-X (not Langerhans cells) histiocytes in the dermis, with a mixed inflammatory component of lymphocytes, neutrophils, plasma cells and eosinophils.

The histiocytes are mainly polyhedral or plump spindle-shaped cells with pale cytoplasm and indistinct cell borders. In mature lesions, foamy histiocytes and Touton giant cells may be prominent, but the early lesions are more monomorphous.

Juvenile xanthogranuloma may present as solitary or multiple papular and nodular lesions up to 10mm in diameter. Most cases occur within the first 9 months of life, but occasional cases occur in adult life. Most lesions involute spontaneously.

8.1.4 **Reticulohistiocytoma** (Figs. 126, 127)

A benign dermal proliferation of large histiocytes with characteristic eosinophilic, finely granular (ground glass) cytoplasm. Lesions may be solitary or multicentric.

In solitary reticulohistiocytoma, there is a dermal nodule composed of large cells with single or multiple ovoid muclei and abundant eosinophilic, granular, periodic acid-Schiff (PAS)-positive cytoplasm. In multicentric reticulohistiocytosis, similar cells are distributed in a more diffuse patterm, singly and in small groups between the collagen bundles of the stroma.

Solitary reticulohistiocytoma presents as a smooth cutaneous nodule. In multicentric reticulohistiocytosis, small cutaneous papules and nodules are associated with arthritis and an increased risk of internal malignancy, occurring most often in middle-aged women.

8.1.5 **Xanthoma** (Fig. 128)

A localized collection of tissue macrophages containing lipid usually arising in response to alteration in serum lipids.

Xanthomas may develop as small lesions on the skin (eruptive xanthoma) or eyelid (xanthelasma), as larger lesions adjacent to the elbow, knee and digits (tuberous xanthoma), within tendons (tendinous xanthoma) or along skin creases (plane xanthoma).

8.2 Malignant

8.2.1 **Atypical fibroxanthoma** (Fig. 129)

A pleomorphic fibrohistiocytic neoplasm of low-grade malignacy. Atypical fibroxanthoma is now regarded as a dermal variant of malignant fibrous histiocytoma.

A nodular dermal tumour with circumscribed borders, confined to the dermis without extension into the subcutis, composed of spindle cells showing pronounced nuclear pleomorphism and hyperchromatism, and giant cells with large, hyperchromatic, single or multiple nuclei including bizarre forms, with plentiful mitoses. The tumours are densely cellular and may extend up to the dermo-epidermal junction, usually without direct continuity with the epidermis, which is elevated and may be ulcerated. Severe solar elastosis and a patchy lymphocytic infiltrate are usually present in the adjacent dermis. The diagnosis is one of exclusion. The lack of direct continuity with the epidermis and negative immunostaining for cytokeratin help to distinguish this neoplasm from spindle cell squamous cell carcinoma. Negative staining for S100 protein and desmin are useful in distinguishing atypical fibroxanthoma from spindle cell melanoma and leiomyosarcoma, respectively.

These tumours characteristically occur on the exposed skin of elderly patients.

8.2.2 Dermatofibrosarcoma protuberans (Fig. 130)

A densely cellular spindle cell tumour of the dermis and subcutis, probably fibrohistiocytic in origin, characterized by a prominent storiform pattern.

The tumour is composed of densely packed, relatively monomorphous, plump spindle cells with low mitotic activity and only moderate nuclear pleomorphism. A prominent storiform (cartwheel or rush mat-like) pattern is present in the densely cellular central areas, whereas at the periphery of the tumour there is diffuse infiltration of the dermal stroma and extension as elongated tendrils into the septa of the panniculus, often producing a characteristic "honeycomb" pattern. The superficial segments of the tumour may resemble neurofibroma or benign fibrous histiocytoma. In contrast to benign fibrous histiocytoma, there is not usually a well-defined, clear subepidermal (grenz) zone, and the epidermis may be attenuated rather than hyperplastic. Immunostaining for CD34 is positive in most cases.

Myxoid areas with a characteristic vascular component composed of slit-like, anastomosing, thin-walled blood vessels with a crow's foot or chicken-wire appearance may be present in some cases. *Bednar tumour* (pigmented dermatofibrosarcoma protuberans, storiform neurofibroma) is a rare variant characterized by a component of melanin-containing spindle cells.

Dermatofibrosarcoma protuberans occurs most frequently on the trunk and proximal extremities, more often in men than women and only rarely in childhood. Initially the tumours form firm plaque-like lesions with red to blue discoloration of the surrounding skin, eventually developing nodules producing the typical protuberant appearance.

8.2.3 Malignant fibrous histiocytoma[1]

8.3 Angiofibromatous proliferations

8.3.1 Adenoma sebaceum (Fig. 131)

A dermal angiofibromatous proliferation associated with tuberous sclerosis.

The epidermis is raised overlying vascular collagenous tissue arranged in concentric layers around hair follicles and vessels, including spindle cells and scattered multinucleated cells. There is no adenomatous proliferation of sebaceous glands; "adenoma sebaceum", therefore, is a misnomer.

Adenoma sebaceum appears in early childhood as symmetrically distributed papules and nodules of the face, particularly the nasolabial groove.

8.3.2 Fibrous papule (Fig. 132)

A benign angiofibromatous lesion of the superficial dermis.

The epidermis is raised in a dome-shaped pattern overlying vascular collagenous tissue in the superficial dermis, containing stellate and multinucleate cells and dilated blood vessels. Melanocytic hyperplasia is frequently present at the dermo-epidermal junction. Positive immunostaining for factor XIIIa in the dermal spindle cells suggests that fibrous papule is a reactive proliferation of dermal dendritic cells rather than a sclerotic melanocytic naevus.

Fibrous papule occurs most often as a solitary papule (3–5 mm in diameter) on the nose of adults.

8.4 Digital mesenchymal tumours

8.4.1 Digital fibroma

A fibroblastic proliferation in the dermis and subcutis of the digits of children.

---

[1] See Weiss SW (1994) Histological typing of soft tissue tumours, WHO International Histological Classification of Tumours, 2nd edn. Springer-Verlag, Berlin Heidelberg New York.

Acanthotic epidermis overlies cellular bands of collagen in which some fibroblasts contain eosinophilic, round or ovoid intracytoplasmic inclusion bodies.

The tumours occur on the toes and fingers of young children and may be present at birth; they are slow growing and tend to recur after excision.

8.4.2 Digital fibrokeratoma

A dermal proliferation of fibroblastic and vascular elements with hyperplasia of the epidermis.

Pronounced acanthosis of the epidermis and elongation of rete ridges overlie dermal proliferation of fibroblasts and small blood vessels in a collagenous stroma.

These lesions are small, firm, exophytic hyperkeratotic nodules of the fingers, toes and, occasionally, the palms and soles of adults.

8.4.3 Digital mucous cyst

A dermal proliferation of mesenchymal cells in a myxoid stroma.

The dermis contains poorly defined zones of connective tissue mucin deposition and proliferation of spindle-shaped and stellate fibroblasts.

Small, solitary nodules develop near the proximal nail fold or on the dorsum of the finger near the distal interphalangeal joint, possibly associated with rupture of an underlying ganglion.

8.5 Dermal mesenchymal tumours of infancy and childhood

A heterogeneous group of rare disorders sharing the features of onset in infancy and childhood and proliferation of mesenchymal elements. This group includes infantile myofibromatosis, fibrous hamartoma of infancy, naevus lipomatosus superficialis, juvenile hyaline fibromatosis and giant cell fibroblastoma.

8.5.1 Infantile myofibromatosis

Dermal nodular aggregates of plump spindle cells resembling smooth muscle are arranged in interlocking fascicles, sometimes with areas of central hyalinization. A characteristic feature is the presence of nodules of tumour cells in a perivascular distribution, forming subendothelial protrusions bulging into the vascular lumina.

8.5.2 Fibrous hamartoma of infancy

In the lower dermis and subcutis, there are thick bands of collagen with fibroblast proliferation, myxoid zones containing groups of small, round and stellate cells resembling embryonic mesenchyme, and lobules of mature fat.

8.5.3 Naevus lipomatosus superficialis

Lobules of mature adipocytes are present in the dermis, representing a form of connective tissue hamartoma.

8.5.4 Juvenile hyaline fibromatosis

Dermal nodules composed of excessive hyalinized collagen.

8.5.5 Giant cell fibroblastoma

Solitary dermal and subcutaneous nodules composed of poorly circumscribed, loosely structured collections of pleomorphic spindle cells in a collagenous or myxoid stroma. Distinctive multinucleated giant cells line cleft-like pseudovascular spaces. The presence of foci resembling dermatofibrosarcoma protuberans suggests that giant cell fibroblastoma may be a juvenile counterpart of that tumour.

8.6 Plexiform fibrohistiocytic tumour

A multinodular tumour of the dermis and subcutis, composed of histiocyte-like cells, fibroblasts and multinucleated giant cells in a plexiform pattern.

Nodules of histiocytic and osteoclast-like giant cells are surrounded by fascicles of fibroblast-like spindle cells intersecting the stroma in a plexiform pattern. Ultrastructural and immunocytochemical studies have indicated histiocytic and myofibroblastic differentiation.

This distinctive lesion is a slowly growing mass of the deep dermis and subcutis, usually in the extremities of children and young adults. Local recurrence is common and regional lymph node metastasis has been described, but visceral metastasis has not been recorded.

9 Nervous Tissue Tumours

9.1 Benign

9.1.1 Neurofibroma[1]

9.1.2 Neurilemoma[1]

9.1.3 Granular cell tumour (Fig. 133)

A benign neoplasm of Schwann cell origin characterized by cells with abundant, coarsely granular cytoplasm.

The tumour is composed of collections of plump cells with abundant, coarsely granular cytoplasm and uniform, central round nuclei. Small collections of these cells are arranged around nerves. In large tumours the cells form dense sheets, with scattered small groups of lymphocytes in the interstitium. The cytoplasmic granules are PAS positive, and immunostaining for S100 protein is strongly positive. The overlying epidermis is often markedly hyperplastic to the extent of pseudoepitheliomatous hyperplasia, especially in tumours of the tongue, anal area and oesophagus.

These neoplasms occur as solitary or multiple symptom-less nodules, most often on the extremities and tongue. The earlier synonym "myoblastoma" is no longer appropriate.

9.1.4 Dermal nerve sheath myxoma and neurothekeoma (Figs. 134, 135)

Benign neoplasms of nerve sheath differentiation with a lobulated architecture, showing variable associated mucinous change.

The tumours are composed of lobules of spindle-shaped and epithelioid cells embedded in a myxoid stroma which is more abundant in tumours composed predominantly of spindle cells. Moderate nuclear pleomorphism and occasional mitoses may be present. Nerve sheath myxoma may represent a variant of neurothekeoma with increased mucin deposition associated with greater age. Accordingly, neurothekeoma may be subdivided into cellular or myxoid variants.

---

[1] Defined as in Weiss SW (1994) Histological typing of soft tissue tumours, WHO International Histological Classification of Tumours. Springe-Verlag, Berlin Heidelberg New York.

Although both variants show positive immunostaining for vimentin, cellular neurothekeoma differs from the classical myxoid tumour by not reacting for S100 protein. This is important in distinguishing cellular neurothekeoma from amelanotic melanoma. These tumours occur most often in young women on the face and upper extremities as solitary nodules.

9.1.5 Palisaded encapsulated neuroma (solitary neuroma) (Fig. 136)

A circumscribed proliferation of axons and supporting cells within the dermis.

These lesions are circumscribed nodular tumours of spindle cells in fascicles surrounded by a thin, perineural connective tissue capsule. The fascicles include axons, Schwann cells and fibroblasts.

These uncommon nodular lesions occur most often on the face of middle-aged patients.

9.1.6 Pacinian neurofibroma (pacinioma) (Fig. 137)

A tumour of the hands and feet composed of corpuscular structures resembling Vater-Pacini corpuscles.

The tumour consists of enlarged, round or ovoid corpuscles composed of multiple concentric lamellae which are sharply circumscribed and embedded in loose fibro-fatty stroma.

Pacinian neurofibroma is a rare tumour presenting usually as a painful nodule of the distal extremities.

9.2 Malignant

9.2.1 Malignant schwannoma[1]

9.2.2 Malignant granular cell tumour (Fig. 138)

A very rare malignant variant of granular cell tumour.

Malignant behaviour is in some cases associated with cytological atypia, showing a transition between benign granular cells and pleomorphic foci, including spindle cells and giant cells with numerous mitoses. In other cases, tumours that his-

---

[1] Defined as in Weiss SW (1994) Histological typing of soft tissue tumours, WHO International Histological Classification of Tumours. Springer-Verlag, Berlin Heidelberg New York.

tologically are typical of benign granular cell tumour may metastasize.

Large size and rapid growth are clinical sings of malignancy.

10 Tumours of Muscle

10.1 Benign

10.1.1 **Piloleiomyoma** (Fig. 139)

A benign neoplasm of arrector pili muscle.

Unlike angioleiomyoma, piloleiomyoma is not sharply circumscribed, consisting of bundles of smooth muscle arranged in an irregular pattern with fibrosis of the intervening stroma.

Piloleiomyomas may be solitary, tender, painful intradermal nodules or multiple smaller nodules arranged in a linear pattern.

10.1.2 **Angioleiomyoma** (Fig. 140)

A benign smooth muscle neoplasm with a prominent vascular component.

The tumour consists of sharply circumscribed dermal and subcutaneous nodules of monomorphic smooth muscle cells with pale cytoplasm and cigar-shaped nuclei with rounded ends. The neoplastic smooth muscle cells merge with the walls of prominent blood vessels of varied size throughout the tumour nodules.

These solitary, painful subcutaneous or intradermal tumours, usually less than 4 cm in diameter, occur most often on the lower extremities.

10.2 Malignant

10.2.1 **Superficial leiomyosarcoma** (Fig. 141)

A malignant neoplasm of smooth muscle cells arising in the dermis.

The tumours are composed of irregular nodules and infiltrating fascicles of smooth muscle cells showing varying degrees of differentiation. Some tumours are monomorphous, composed of smooth muscle cells with hyperchromatic nuclei and scattered mitoses, whereas other zones may be pleomorphic, including bizarre cells with giant nuclei and numerous mitoses. Positive immunostaining for desmin and smooth muscle actin is helpful in distinguishing leiomyosarcoma from other spindle cell tumours.

Dermal leiomyosarcomas are solitary, firm nodules less than 2 cm in diameter and are usually asymptomatic. Metastasis is rare and the prognosis is usually favourable.

11 Miscellaneous Tumours

11.1 Primary cutaneous neuroendocrine carcinoma (Merkel cell tumour) (Fig. 142)

A highly malignant neoplasm of poorly differentiated cells showing epithelial and neuroendocrine features.

These tumours are composed of dense sheets and strands of generally monomorphic cells, sometimes with a prominent trabecular pattern, usually separated from the epidermis by a narrow clear zone. Foci of epidermal involvement in a minority of cases suggest invasion from the underlying tumour mass rather than intra-epidermal origin. The cells are larger than lymphocytes with round or ovoid, deeply basophilic nuclei, small inconspicuous nucleoli and a finely dispersed granular chromatin pattern. The cytoplasm is usually scanty and eosinophilic or basophilic, but occasionally it is more abundant and paler staining. Nuclear moulding produces a "ball in mit" pattern as a frequent finding, mitotic figures are abundant and necrosis occurs in scattered individual cells and segments of tumour. Extracellular mucin is often seen in the stroma, and lymphatic invasion is frequently present. The adjacent dermal stroma often shows severe solar elastosis; concurrent solar keratosis, lentigo maligna and in situ squamous cell carcinoma have been noted in the overlying epidermis in a small proportion of cases. Although mainly monomorphic, the tumours frequently include foci of cellular pleomorphism with occasional giant nuclei; foci of squamous and glandular differentiation also occur.

The differential diagnosis includes lymphoma, metastatic small cell carcinoma and melanoma. The morphology in routine histological sections, especially the growth pattern and the nuclear characteristics, provides helpful diagnostic criteria, but the characteristic immunocytochemical findings of paranuclear cytokeratin globules and positivity for neurone-specific enolase, and the ultrastructural demonstration of neuroendocrine granules indicate neuroendocrine differentiation. These findings, however, do not exclude metastatic small cell carcinoma, especially of bronchial origin, which have similar immunocytochemical and ultrastructural features. The presence of foci of squamous and glandular epithelium in some cases, their cytokeratin positivity and the dermal situation of most tumours suggest that they might be derived from epithelium, possibly adnexal, rather than from Merkel cells.

Cutaneous neuroendocrine carcinomas occur mainly on sun-exposed skin in elderly patients, presenting as smooth, occasionally ulcerated, nodular masses.

11.2 **Epithelioid sarcoma** (Fig. 143)

A distinctive malignant soft tissue neoplasm of cytokeratin-positive epithelioid and spindle cells.

The tumour is composed of irregular nodules of the characteristic epithelioid cells with eosinophilic cytoplasm and pleomorphic nuclei, merging with spindle cells. A patchy lymphocytic infiltrate may be seen in and around the tumour nodules with focal haemorrhage and haemosiderin deposition. Mitoses are present in varied numbers, and vascular invasion is a common feature. The low-power appearances can resemble rheumatoid nodule and granuloma annulare, where sharply defined central zones of necrosis and degeneration, often with deposition of mucin, are surrounded by neoplastic cells. The necrosis is often present in the centres of dense aggregates of tumour cells, however, and not only in collagen, as seen in benign necrobiotic conditions. The epithelioid and spindle cells of the neoplasm do not produce the distinctly biphasic or pseudoglandular pattern of synovial sarcoma, but the growth pattern may resemble angiosarcoma, where epithelioid cells line cleft-like spaces between collagen bundles.

Immunostaining for cytokeratin and vimentin is usually strongly positive, whereas staining for epithelial membrane antigen is variable. Ultrastructural features include cytoplasmic intermediate filaments and intercellular junctions. The histogenesis is still obscure, however, although synovial and primitive mesenchymal origins have been suggested. This neoplasm most commonly occurs as ulcerating nodules of the skin and soft tissues of the distal extremities, more often in male than in female patients. It may be confused clinically and histologically with a variety of benign granulomatous processes, such as granuloma annulare and rheumatoid nodule, and with other neoplasms, such as synovial sarcoma, angiosarcoma, malignant melanoma and spindle cell squamous cell carcinoma.

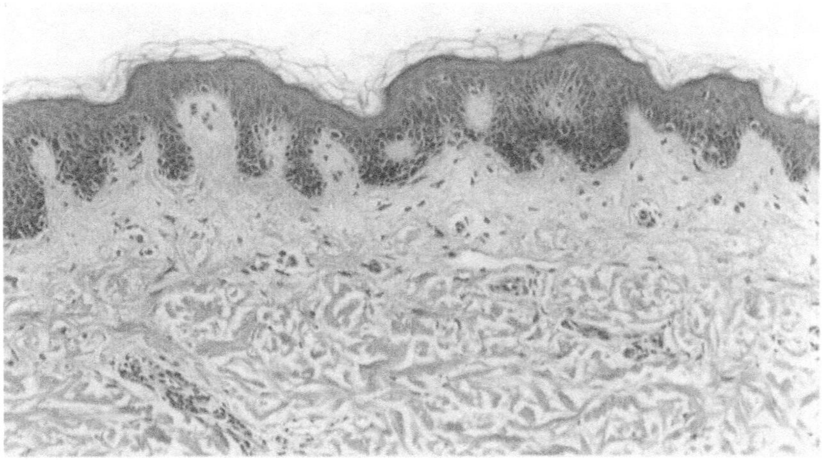

Fig. 1. *Lentigo simplex.* Elongated rete ridges, hyperpigmentation of the basal layer and increase in number of enlarged melanocytes arranged singly along the basal layer

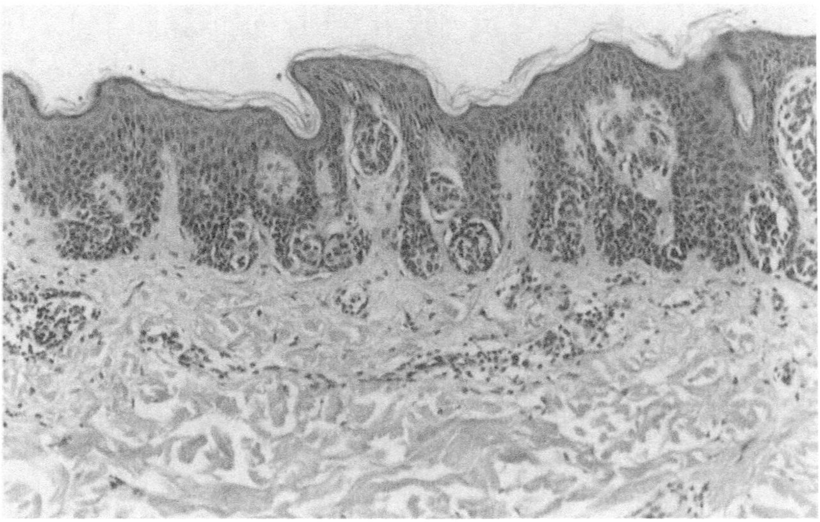

Fig. 2. *Junctional melanocytic naevus.* Nests of melanocytes are present at the dermo-epidermal junction, predominantly at the bases of elongated rete ridges

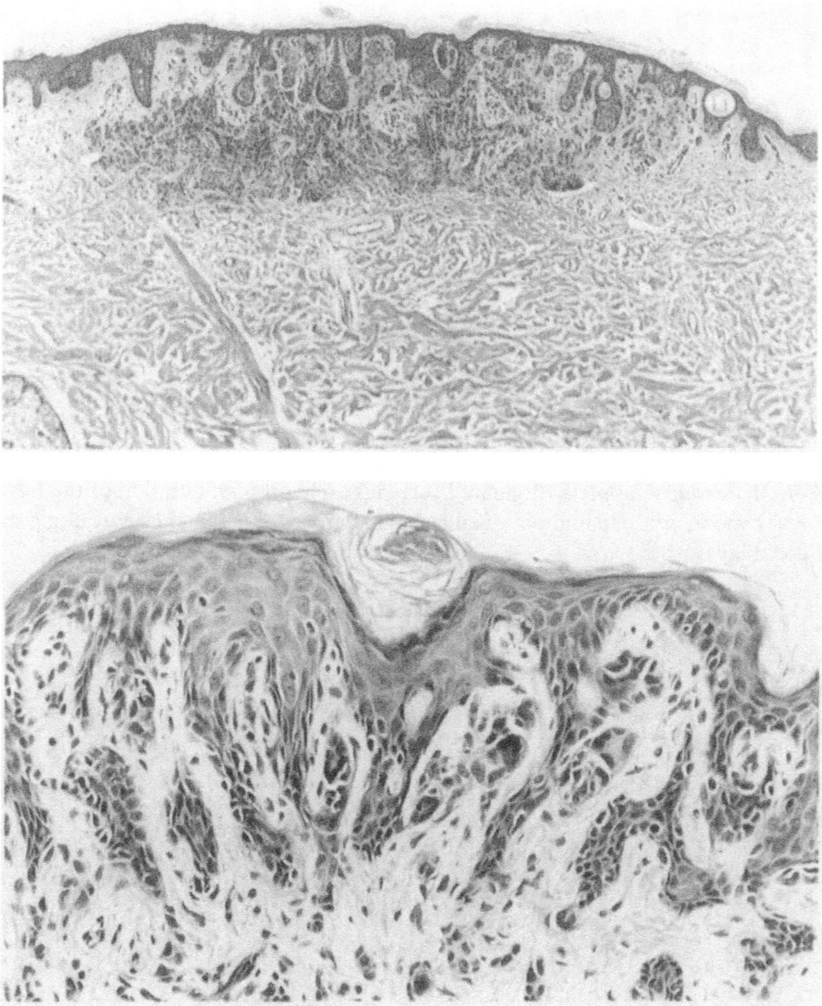

a

b

Fig. 3a,b. *Compound melanocytic naevus.* **a** Nests of melanocytes in the dermis as well as the dermo-epidermal junction, smaller and more diffusely arranged in the deeper dermis. **b** The nests of melanocytes include multinucleated giant cells

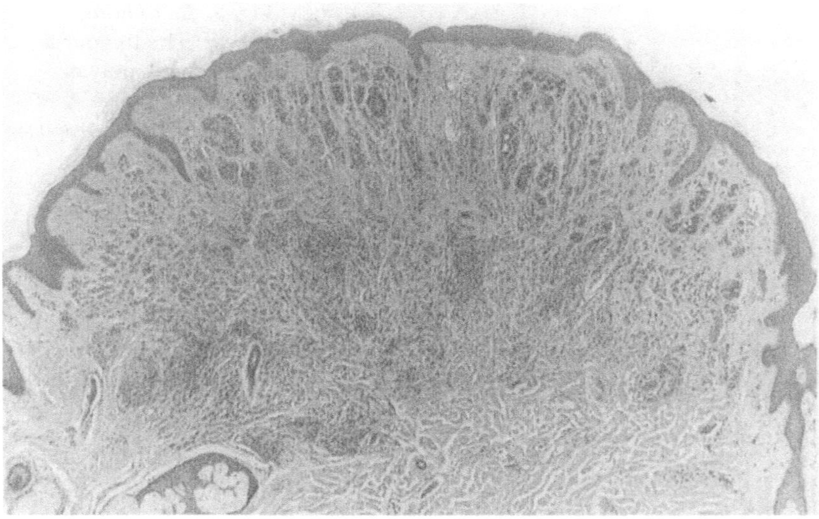

Fig. 4. *Dermal melanocytic naevus.* Entirely intradermal tumour in a nested pattern in the superficial layers, composed of small naevoid melanocytes in the deep dermis

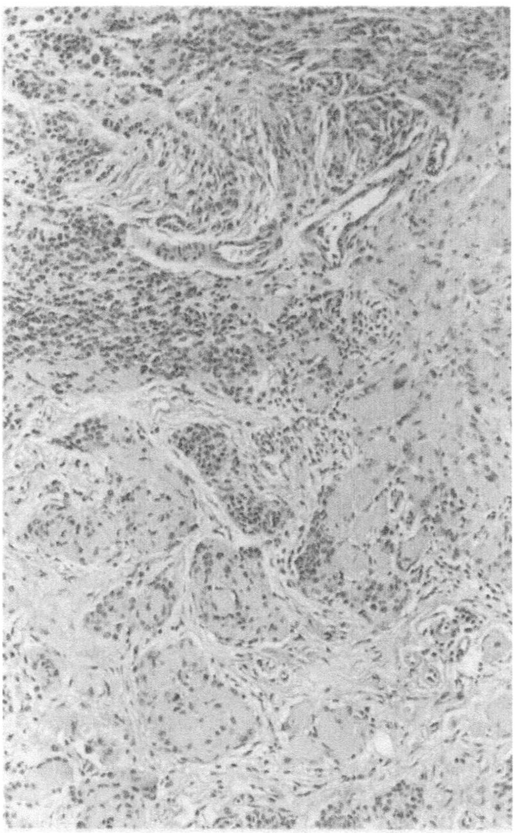

Fig. 5. *Dermal melanocytic naevus.* The deeper layers of this dermal melanocytic naevus include neuroid structures similar to Wagner-Meissner corpuscles (neuroid dermal melanocytic naevus)

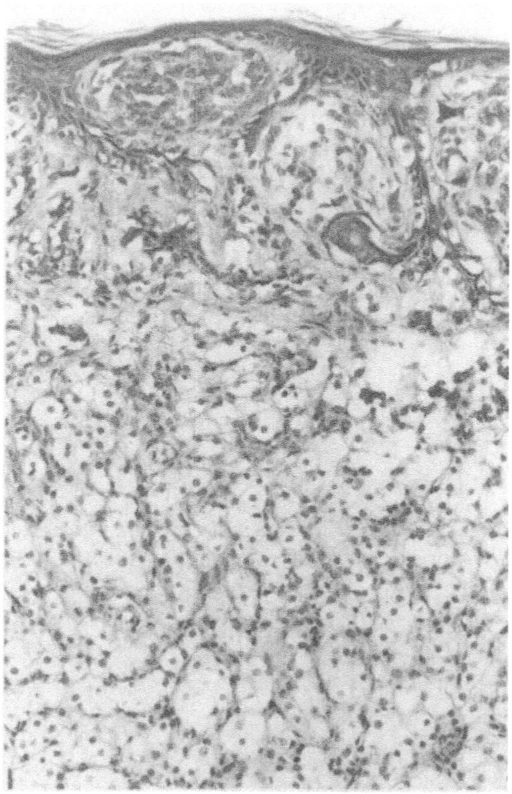

Fig. 6. *Balloon cell naevus.* The tumour is composed mainly of melanocytes with abundant clear cytoplasm and central nuclei

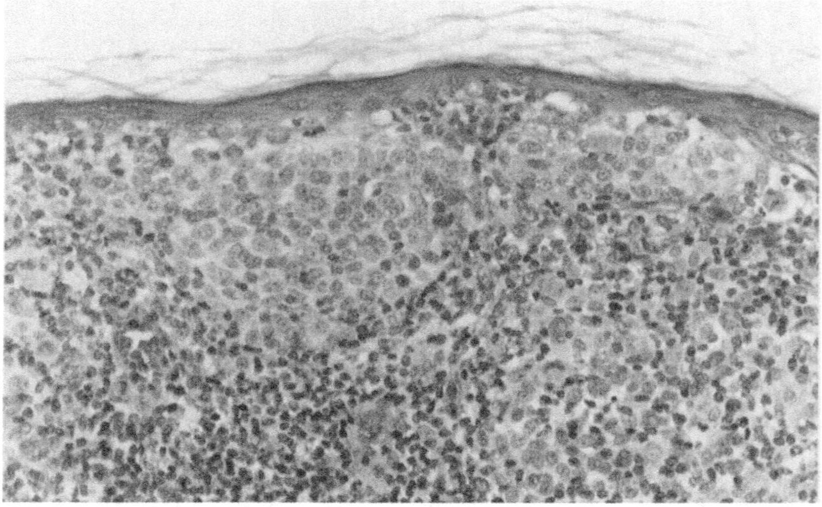

Fig. 7. *Halo naevus.* Compound naevus with a dense lymphocytic infiltrate between the naevoid melanocytes of the dermal component

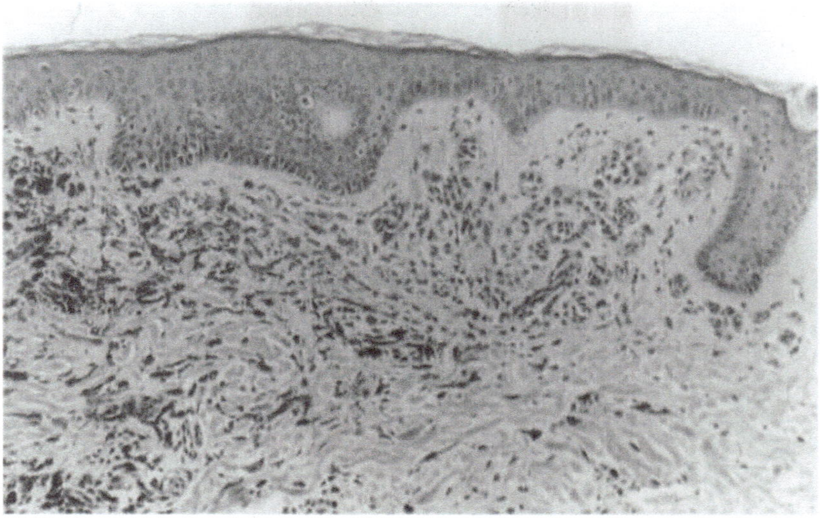

Fig. 8. *Combined intradermal naevus and blue naevus.* Nests of epithelioid naevus cells in the dermis (*right*) and heavily pigmented spindle and dendritic cells arranged between collagen bundles in the adjacent stroma (*left*)

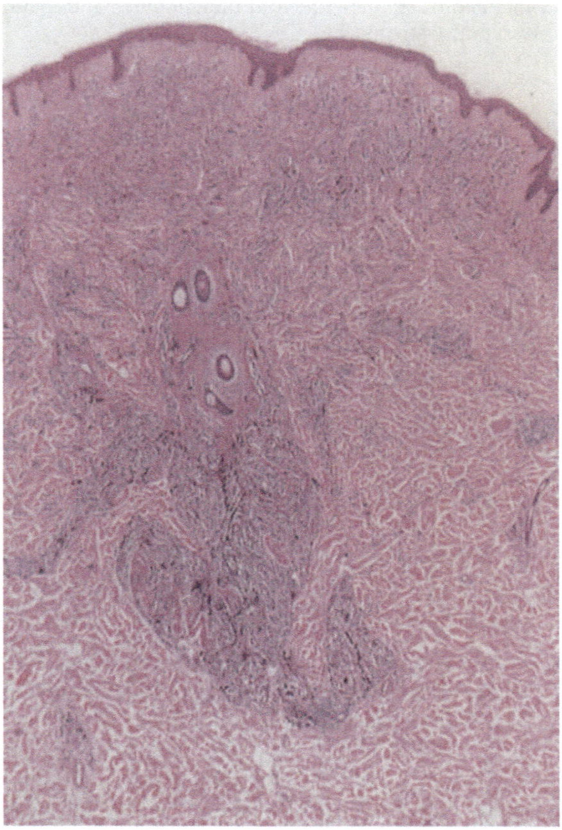

Fig. 9a. *Deep penetrating naevus.* A wedge-shaped lesion composed of irregular collections of variably pigmented cells extending into the deep dermis.

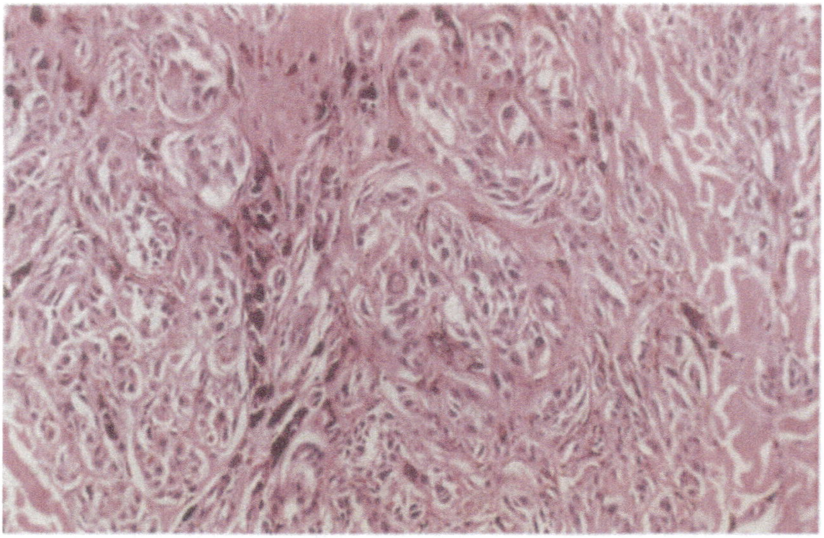

Fig. 9b. *Deep penetrating naevus.* In the deep dermis the lesion includes large cells with nuclear pseudo-inclusions, smaller naevoid melanocytes and groups of melanophages in the intervening stroma

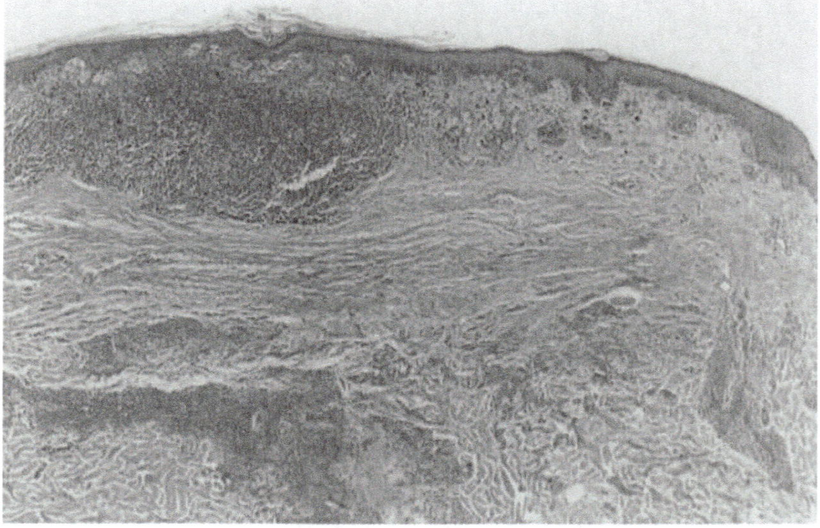

Fig. 10a. *Recurrent melanocytic naevus (pseudomelanoma).* Residual deep dermal naevus is separated by a zone of scarring from a more superficial compound naevus including nests of varied size at the junction.

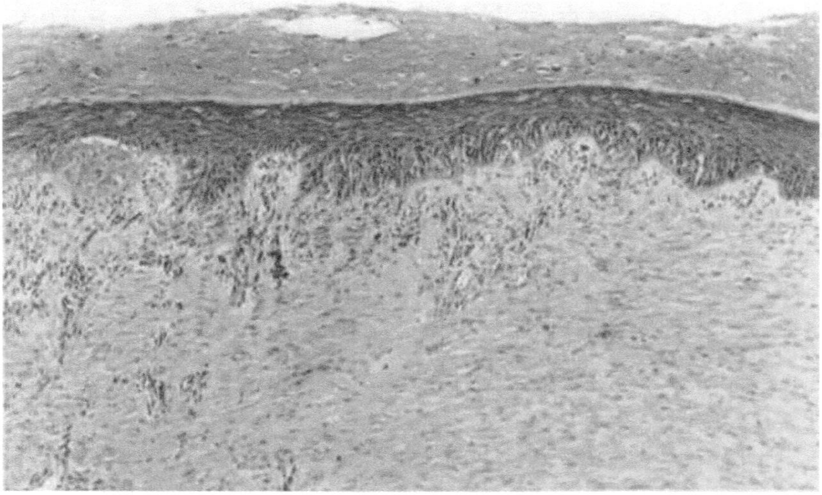

Fig. 10b. *Recurrent melanocytic naevus (pseudomelanoma).* A zone of cellular scarring in the superficial dermis is surmounted by irregular nests of junctional naevus cells with scattered single melanocytes above the basal layer and pigmentation in the stratum corneum

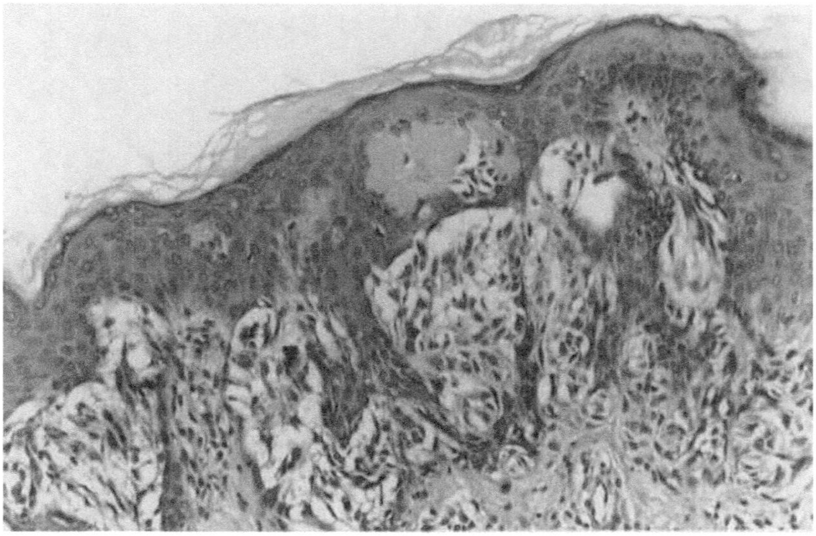

Fig. 11. *Spitz naevus.* Amorphous globoid (Kamino) bodies are present in the epidermis and at the dermo-epidermal junction overlying nests of epithelioid and spindle cells with peripheral cleavage

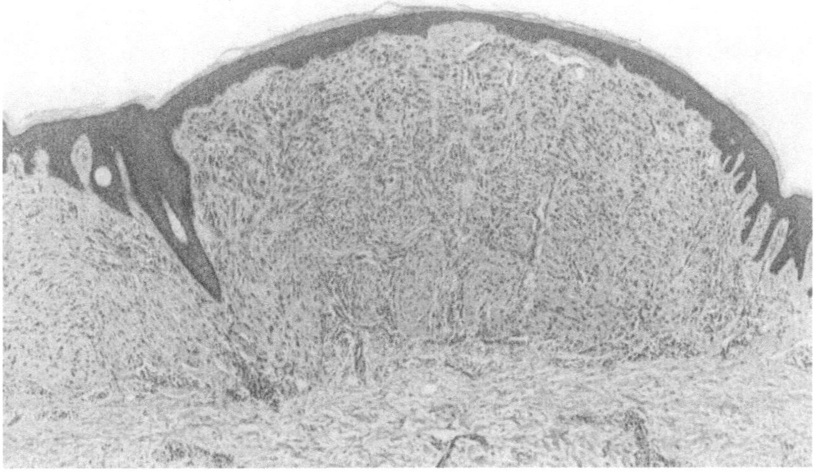
a

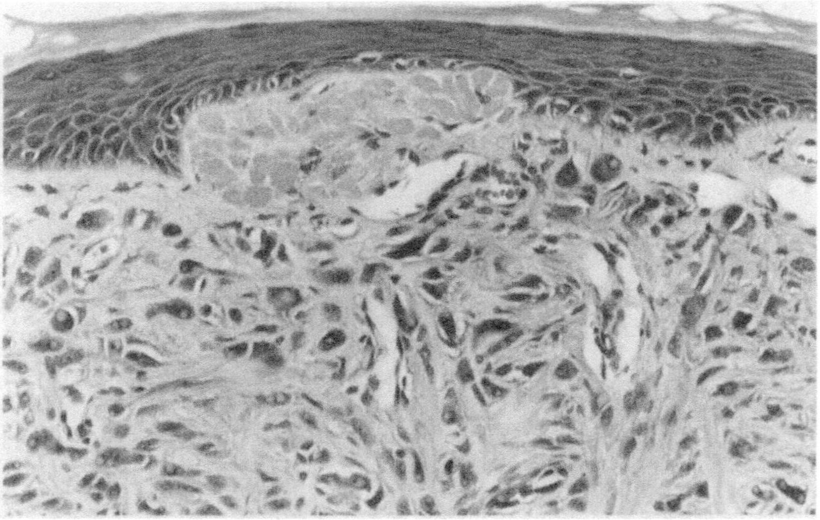
b

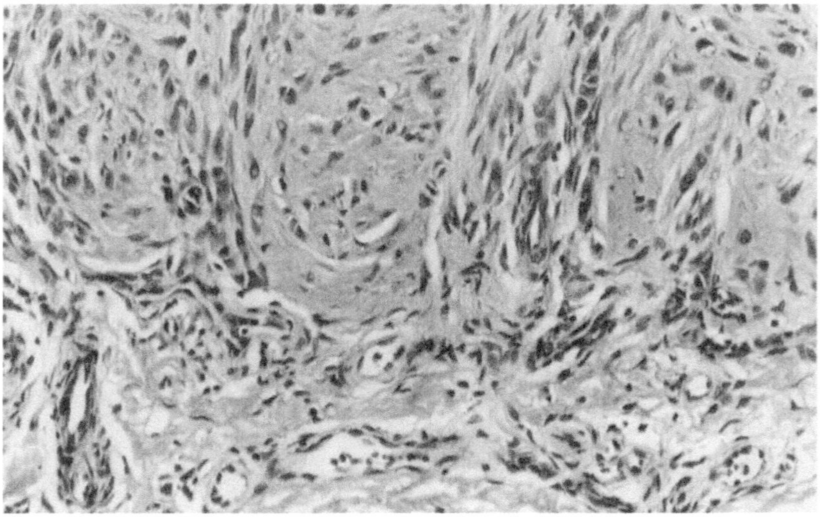
c

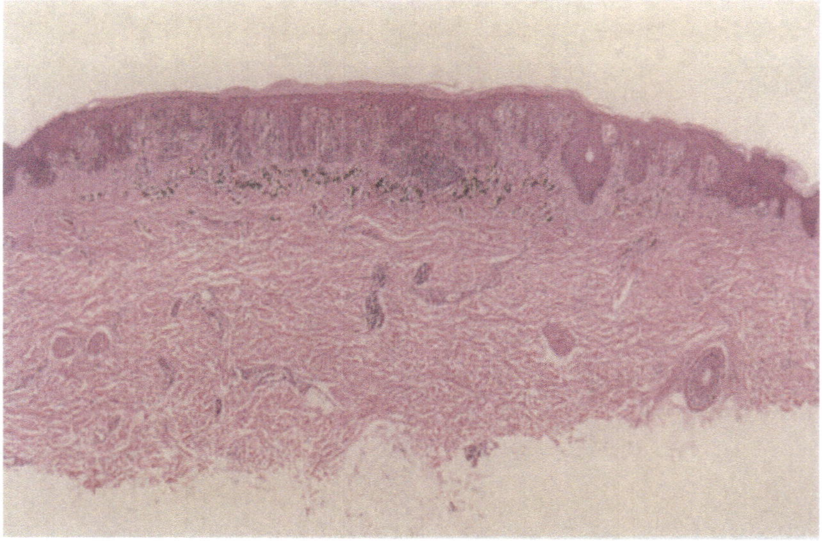

a

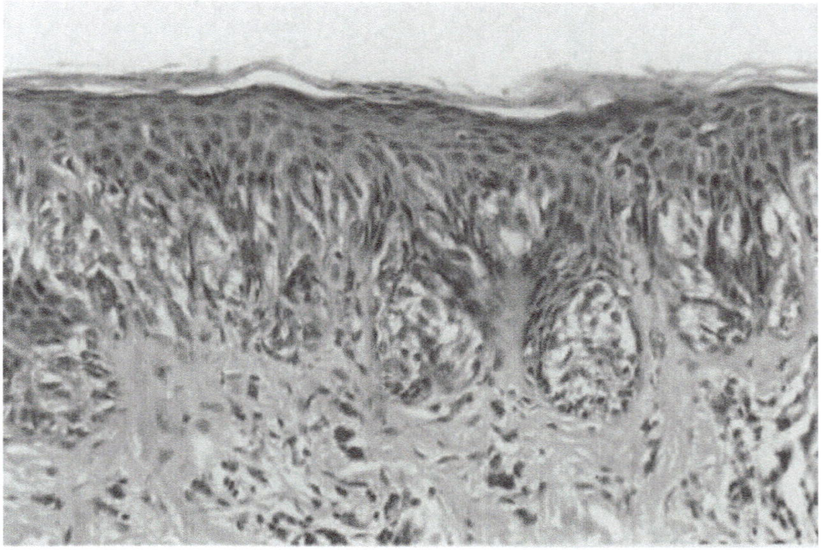

b

Fig. 13a,b. *Pigmented spindle cell naevus of Reed.* **a** A sharply circumscribed, symmetrical melanocytic lesion. **b** Nests of heavily pigmented spindle cells at the dermo-epidermal junction and in the papillary dermis

Fig. 12a–c. *Dermal Spitz naevus.* **a** Circumscribed, symmetrical intradermal tumour. **b** Large epithelioid melanocytes with intranuclear cytoplasmic invaginations arranged singly and in small groups in collagenous stroma with cytoid bodies in the papillary dermis. **c** At the base of the lesion in the deep reticular dermis, the naevoid melanocytes are much smaller, indicating maturation; single cells are dispersed between collagen bundles

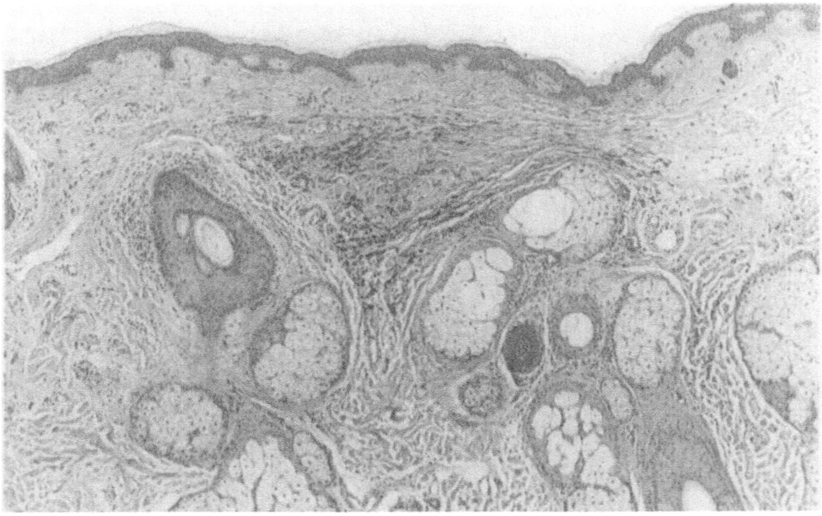

a

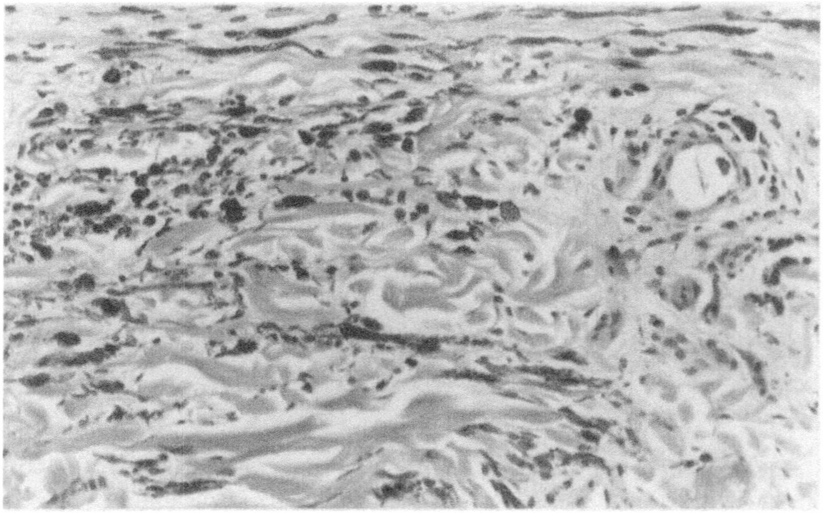

b

Fig. 14a,b. *Common blue naevus.* **a** A poorly defined pigmented lesion in the reticular dermis. **b** Heavily pigmented dendritic and spindle-shaped melanocytes arranged in splayed pattern between the collagen bundles

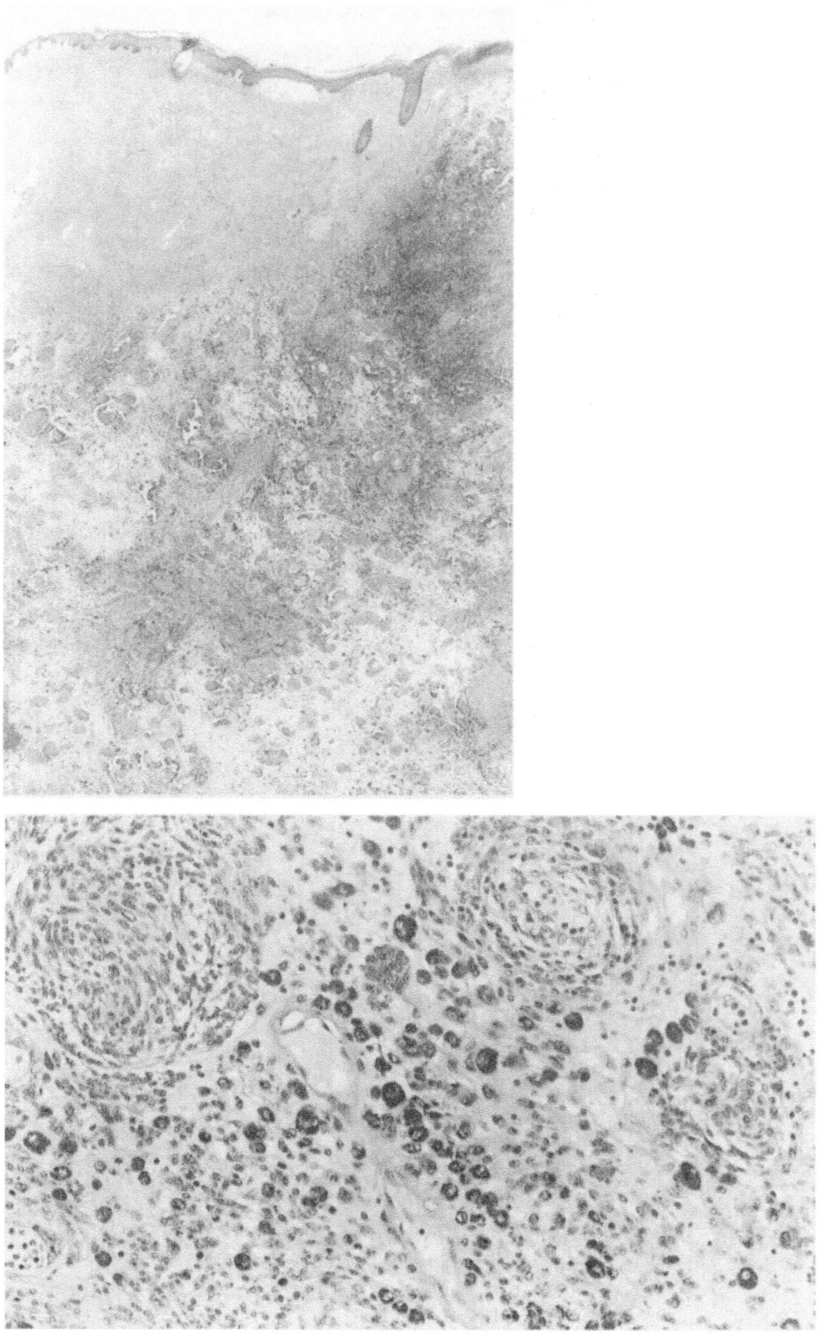

a

b

Fig. 15a,b. *Cellular blue naevus.* **a** A large tumour expanding the reticular dermis and extending into the subcutis, showing a biphasic growth pattern in the deeper layers. **b** A biphasic growth pattern marked by alveolar clusters of clear cells and a more diffuse array of heavily pigmented epithelioid and spindle cells

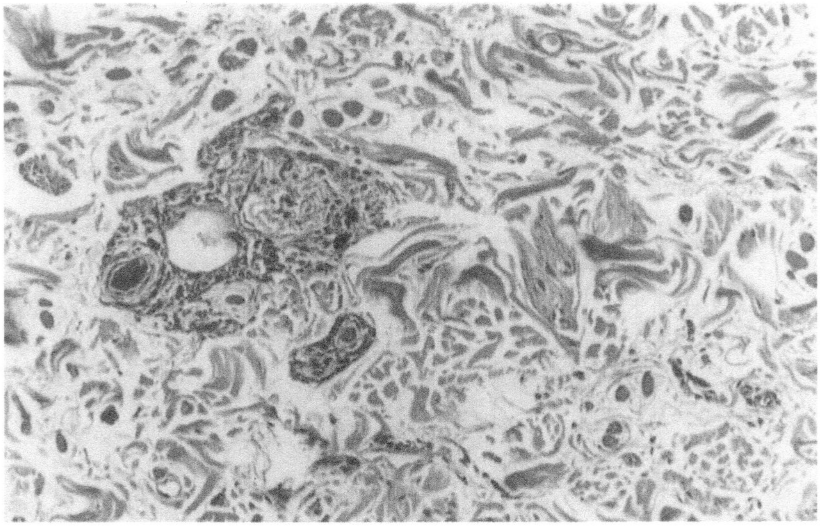

Fig. 16. *Naevus of Ota.* Dendritic and spindle-shaped melanocytes arranged around blood vessels and nerves of the reticular dermis

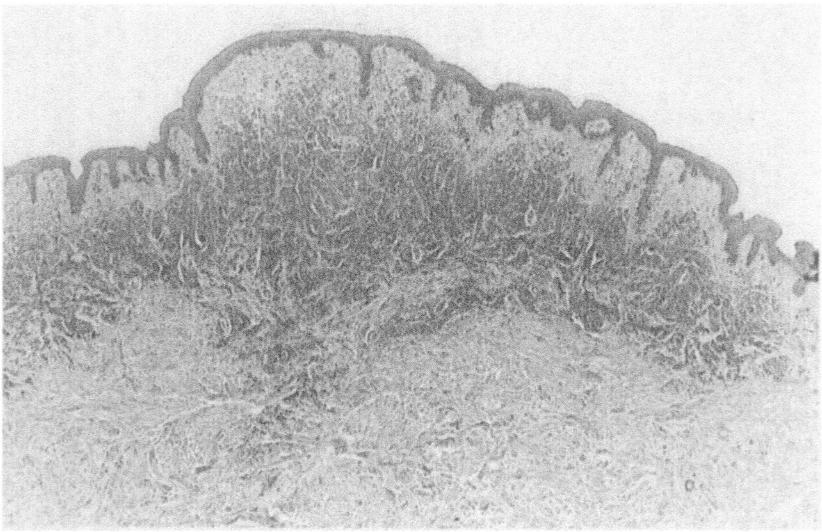

Fig. 17a. *Small congenital naevus.* Compound naevus with groups of small naevus cells extending into the deep reticular dermis.

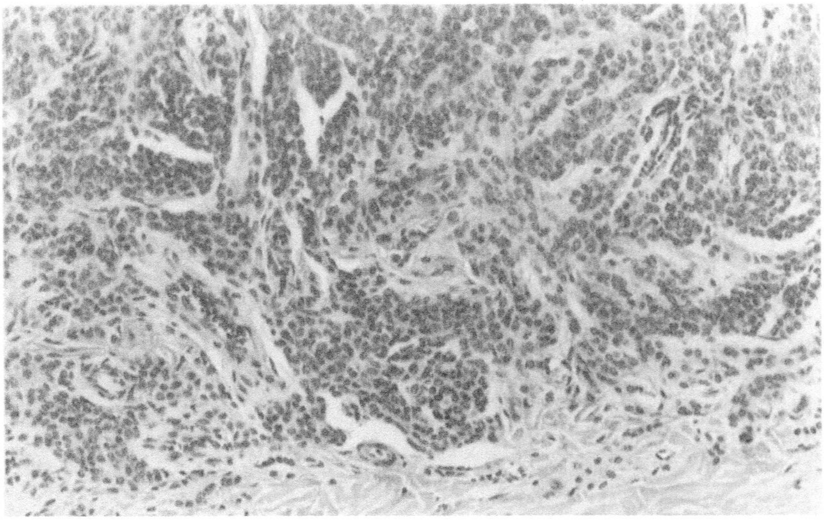

Fig. 17b. *Small congenital naevus.* Small naevus cells arranged around blood vessels in the reticular dermis

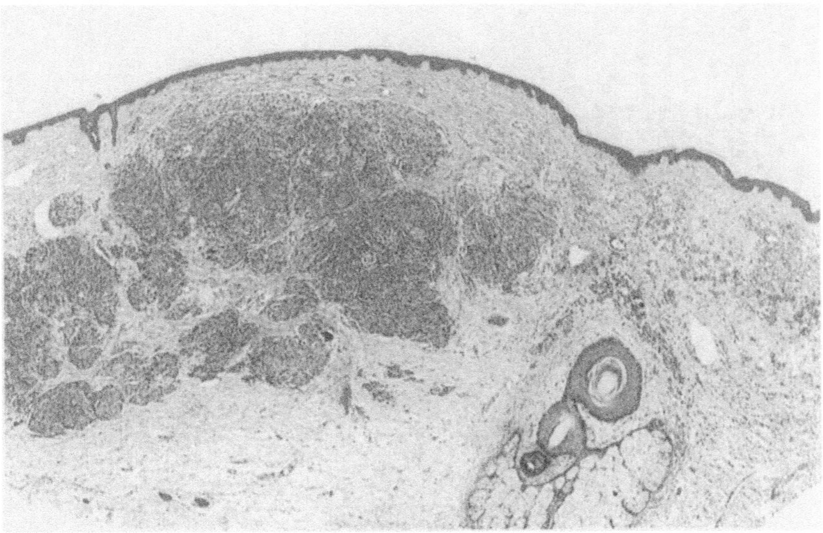

Fig. 18a. *Proliferative nodules in giant congenital naevus.* Densely cellular nodules blend with less cellular dermal congenital naevus (*right*)

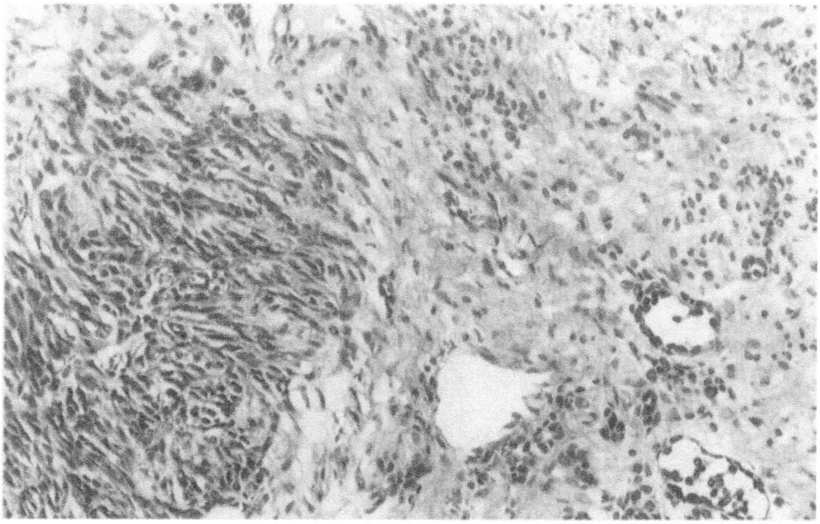

Fig. 18b. *Proliferative nodules in giant congenital naevus.* Spindle cell nodule (*left*); loosely structured dermal congenital naevus in vascular stroma (*right*)

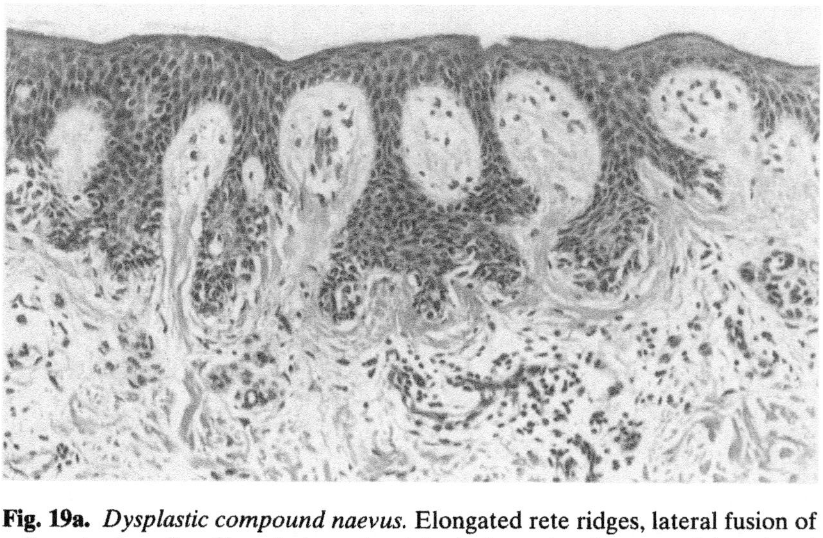

Fig. 19a. *Dysplastic compound naevus.* Elongated rete ridges, lateral fusion of cell nests, lamellar fibroplasia and cytological atypia of scattered junctional melanocytes (random cytological atypia)

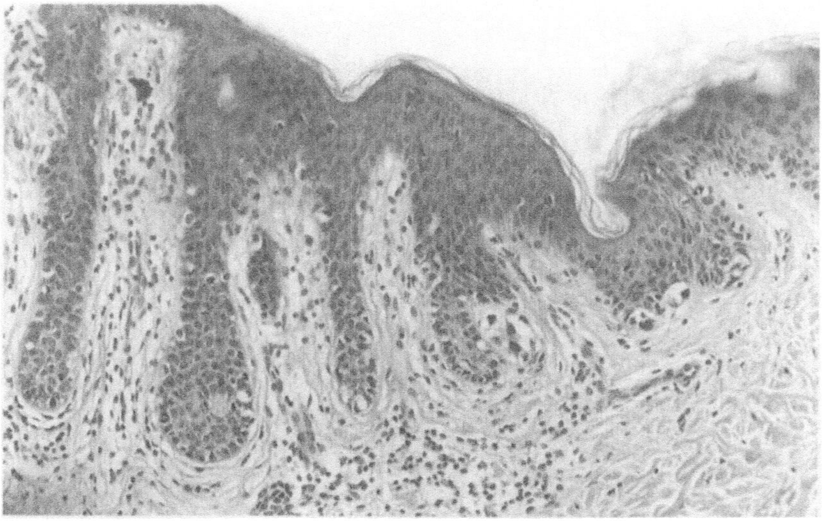

Fig. 19b. *Dysplastic compound naevus.* Elongated rete ridges, lamellar fibroplasia, a sparse lymphocytic infiltrate in the superficial dermis and random cytological atypia of junctional melanocytes

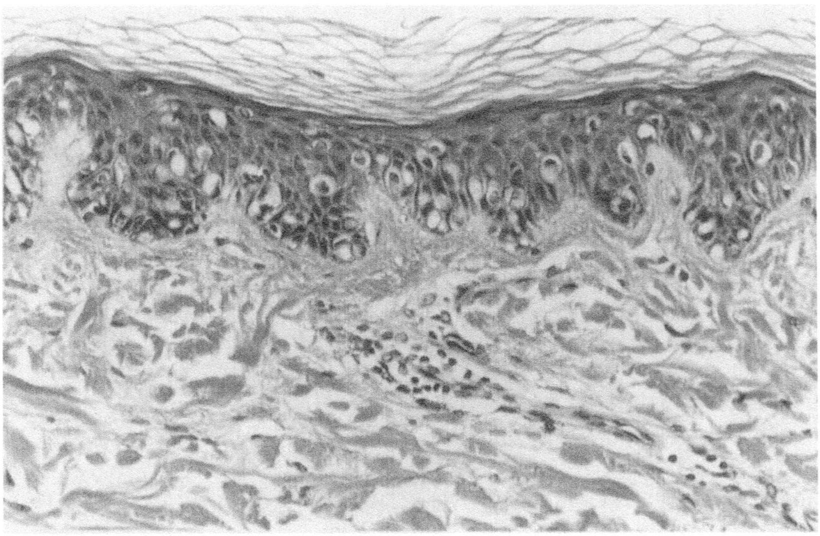

Fig. 20. *Superficial spreading melanoma, in situ.* Atypical epithelioid cells distributed throughout the epidermis with single cells predominating over small nests

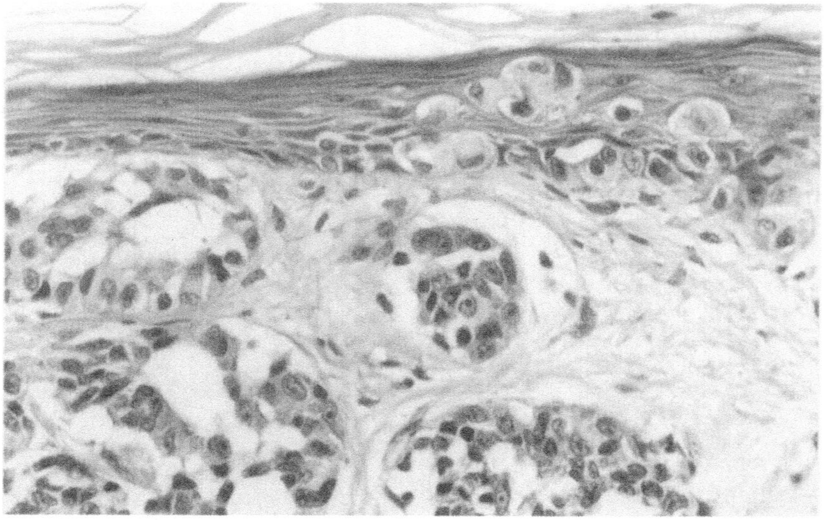

Fig. 21. *Superficial spreading melanoma.* Pagetoid infiltration of the epidermis by atypical epithelioid melanocytes singly and in irregular nests, with invasion of the underlying papillary dermis

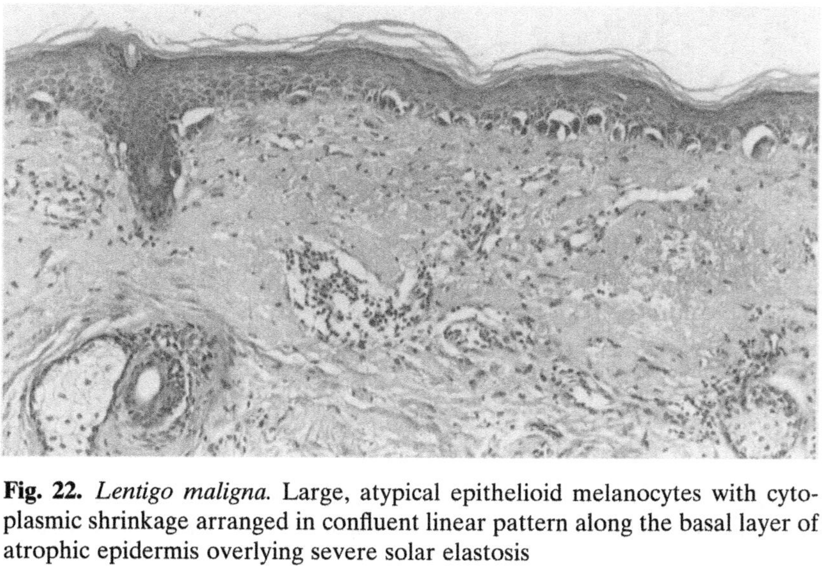

Fig. 22. *Lentigo maligna.* Large, atypical epithelioid melanocytes with cytoplasmic shrinkage arranged in confluent linear pattern along the basal layer of atrophic epidermis overlying severe solar elastosis

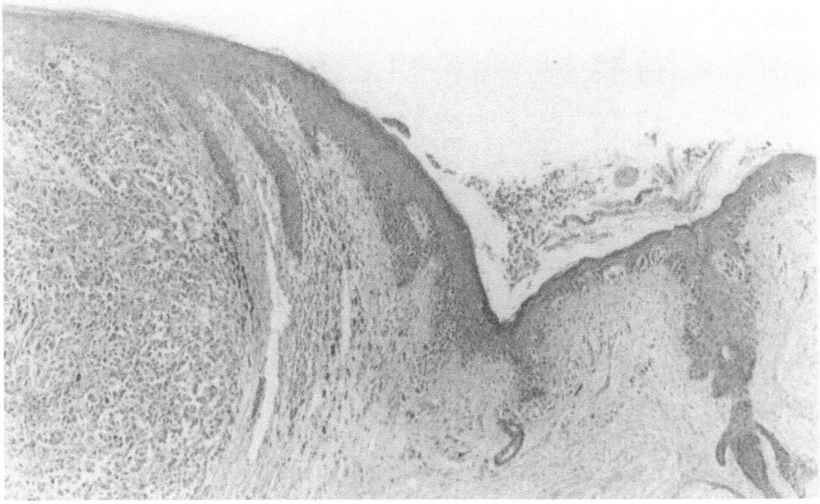

Fig. 23. *Lentigo maligna melanoma.* An invasive nodule of atypical melanocytes extends into the reticular dermis, with an extensive adjacent intraepidermal component of the lentigo maligna type

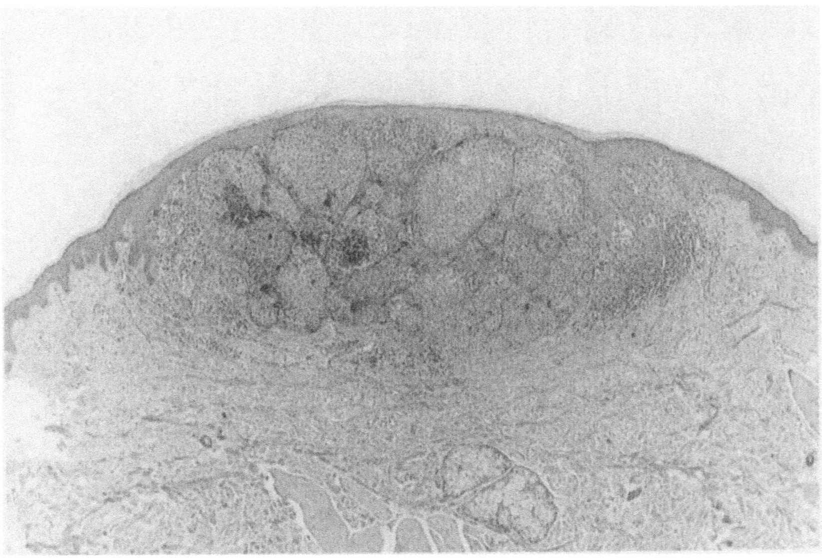

Fig. 24a. *Nodular melanoma.* A solid nodule of atypical epithelioid melanocytes invading the reticular dermis

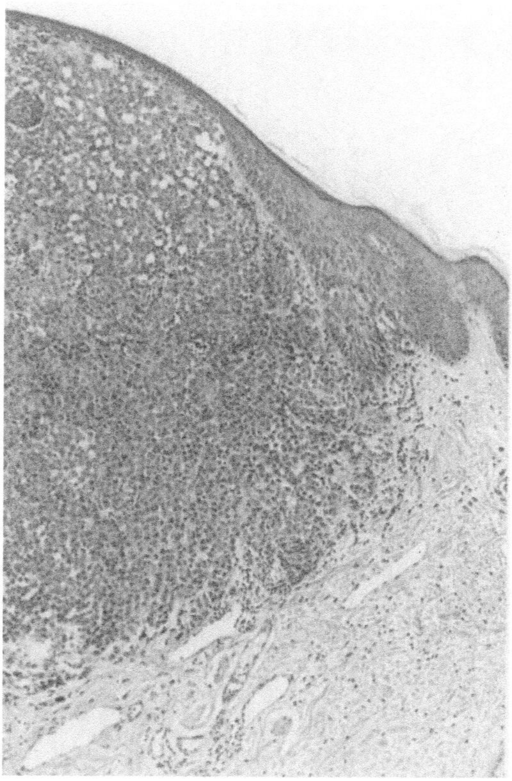

Fig. 24b. *Nodular melanoma.* There is no adjacent intra-epidermal component

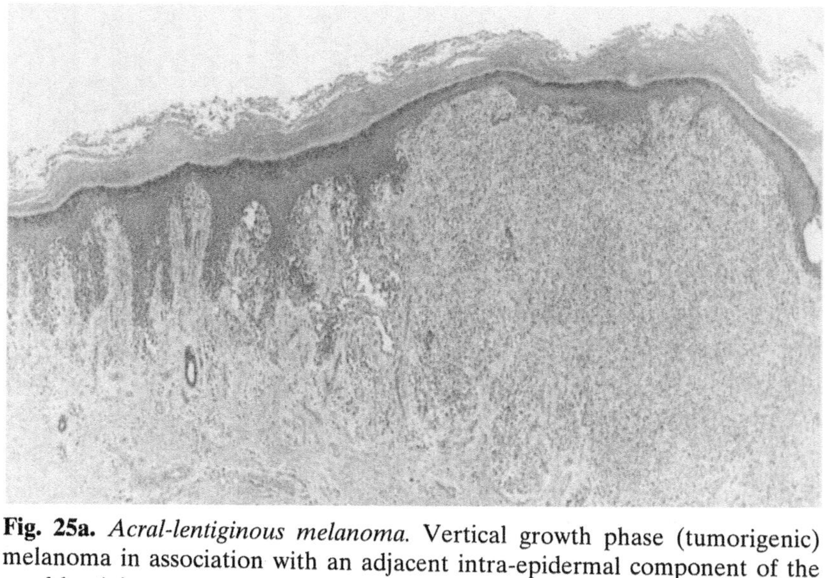

Fig. 25a. *Acral-lentiginous melanoma.* Vertical growth phase (tumorigenic) melanoma in association with an adjacent intra-epidermal component of the acral-lentiginous type

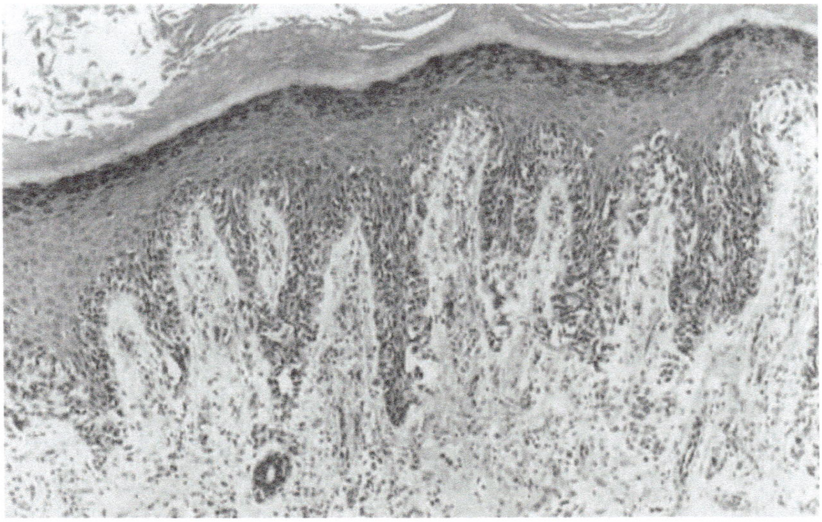

Fig. 25b. *Acral-lentiginous melanoma.* Hyperplastic epidermis with elongated rete ridges; atypical epithelioid melanocytes in a confluent linear pattern along the basal layer and extending up into the lower third of the epidermis

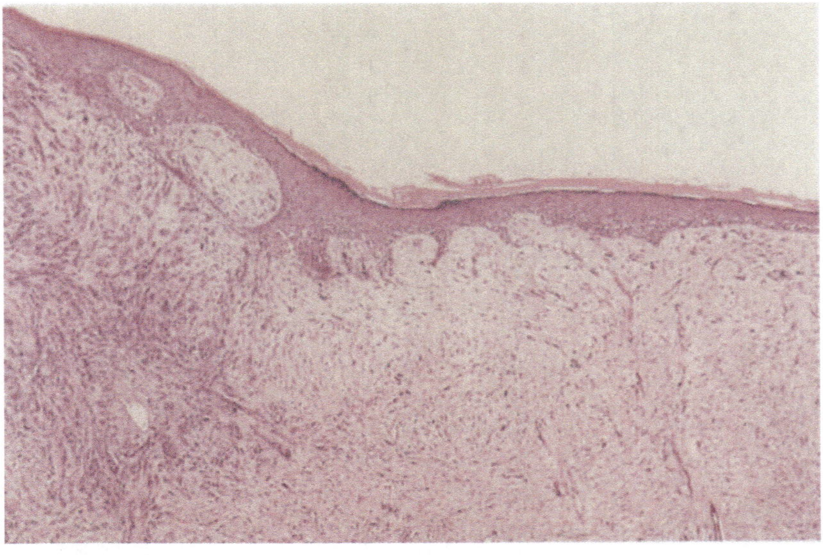

Fig. 26a. *Desmoplastic melanoma.* Atypical lentiginous melanocytic proliferation overlies atypical spindle cells in sparse (*right*) and denser distribution (*left*).

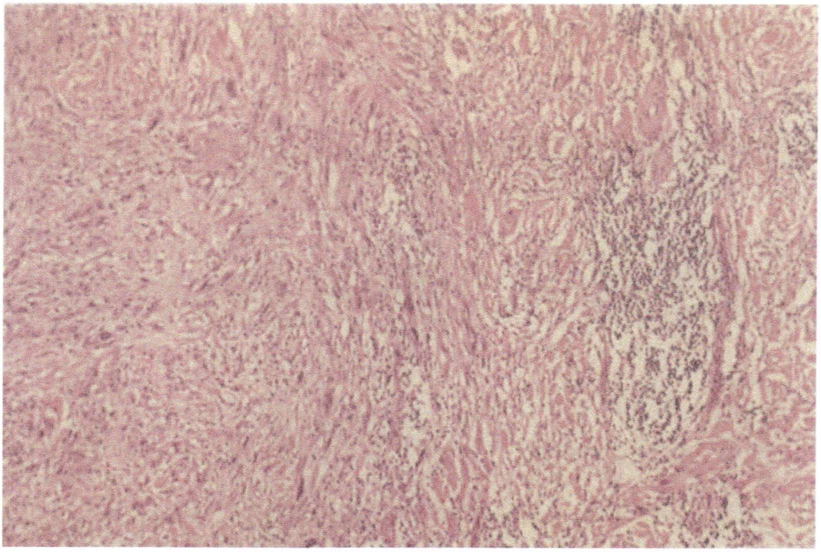

b

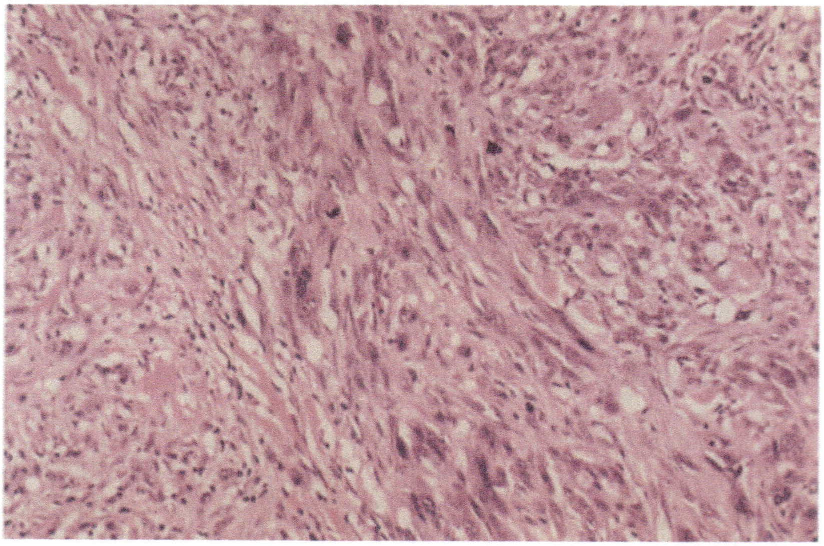

c

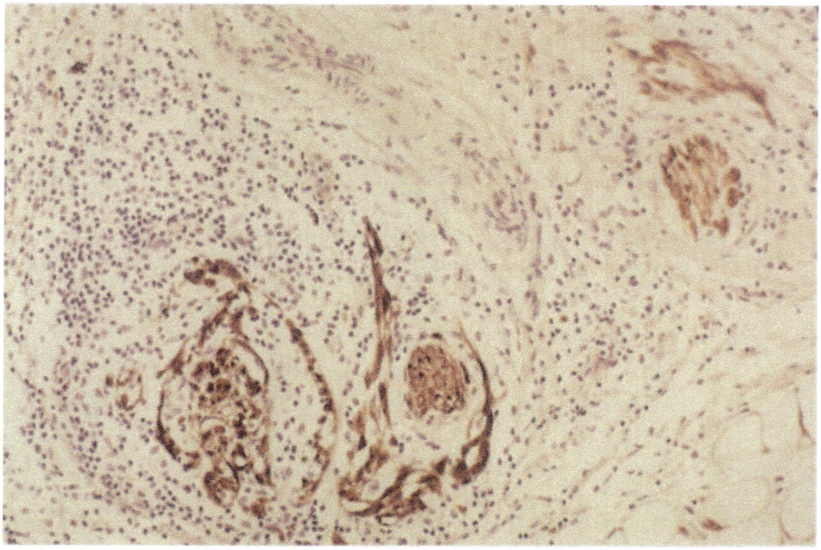

d

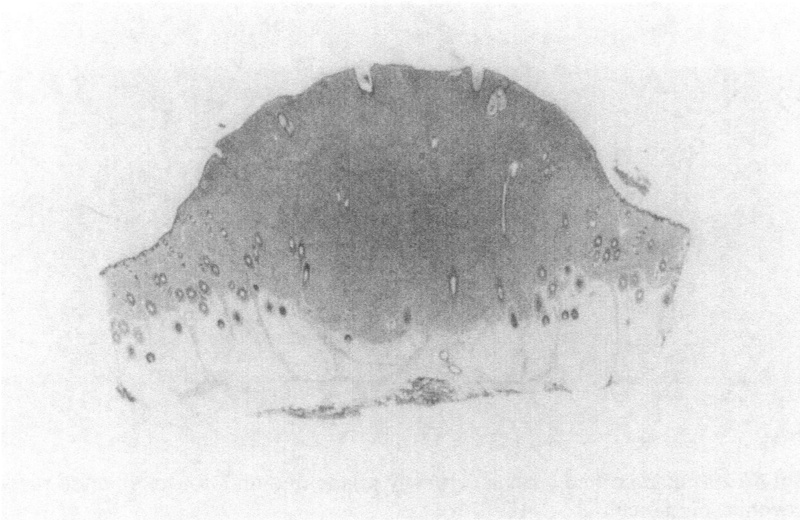

a

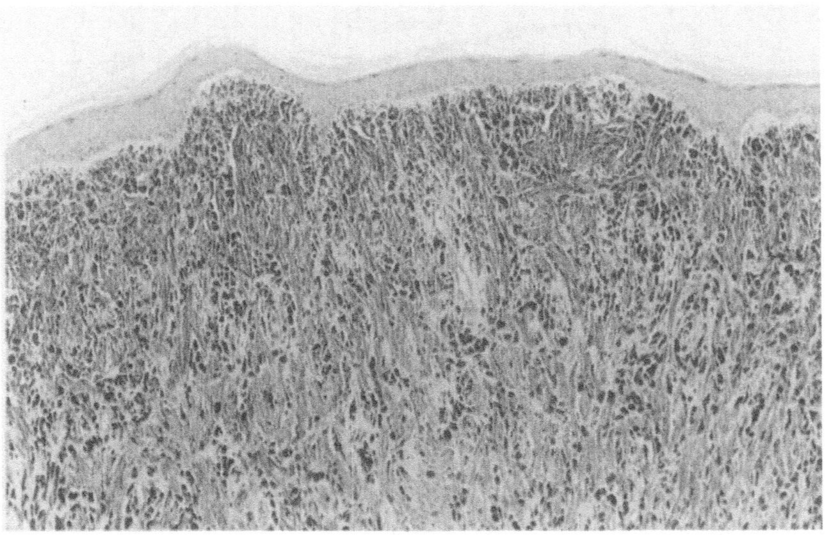

b

Fig. 27a,b. *Malignant blue naevus.* The lesion forms a large nodule bulging into the subcutis. The epidermis is separated by a narrow clear zone from the densely cellular dermal tumour composed mainly of spindle cells, without the biphasic growth pattern typical of cellular blue naevus

◀

Fig. 26b–d. *Desmoplastic melanoma.* **b** A patchy lymphocytic infiltrate separates fascicles of atypical spindle cells arranged perpendicular to the epidermis. **c** In a more cellular zone the spindle cells show nuclear pleomorphism and several mitoses. **d** Positive immunostaining for S100 protein in atypical spindle cells infiltrating nerve bundles in the dermis

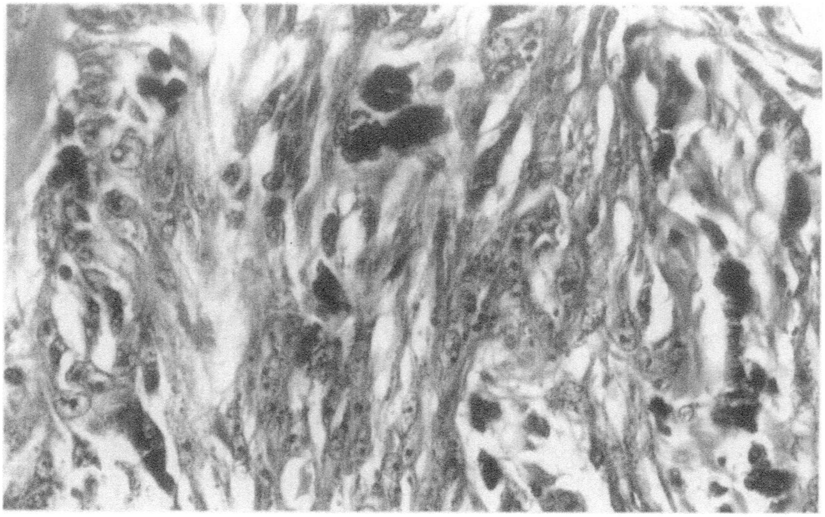

Fig. 27c. *Malignant blue naevus.* Heavily pigmented and non-pigmented pleomorphic spindle cells

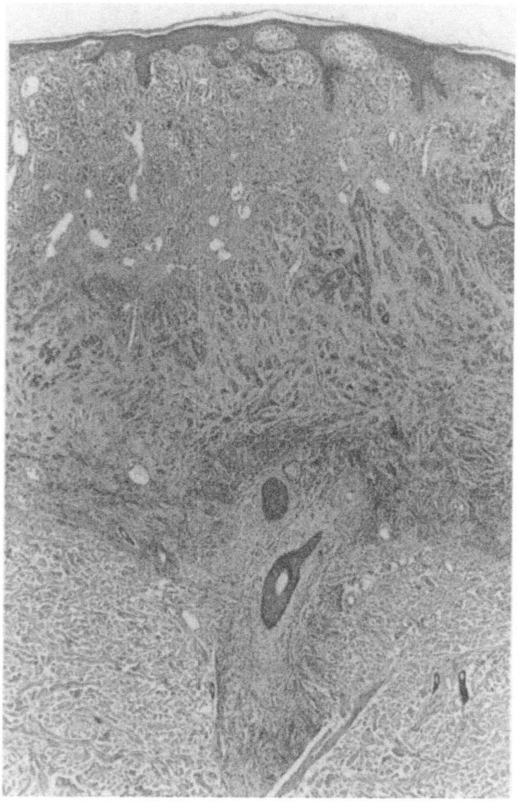

Fig. 28a. *Superficial spreading melanoma in congenital naevus in an adult.* Superficial spreading melanoma overlies residual congenital naevus extending into the deep reticular dermis.

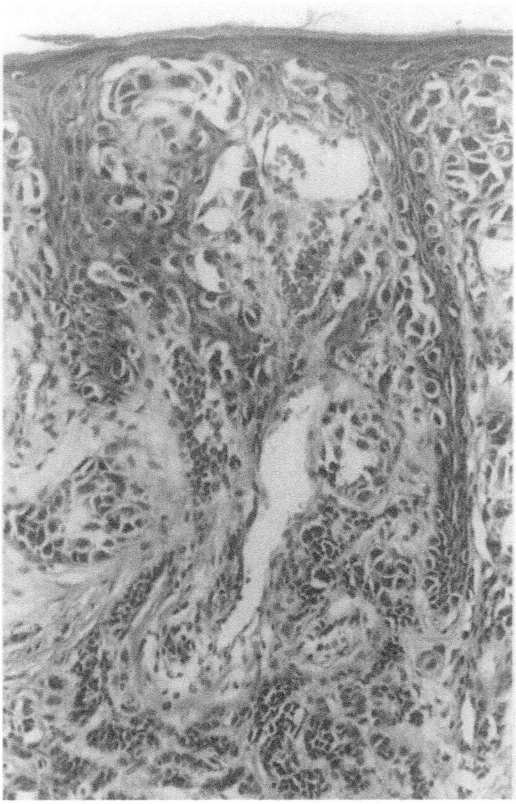

Fig. 28b. *Superficial spreading melanoma in congenital naevus in an adult.* Atypical melanocytes in a pagetoid pattern in the epidermis and invading the papillary dermis overlying residual naevoid melanocytes

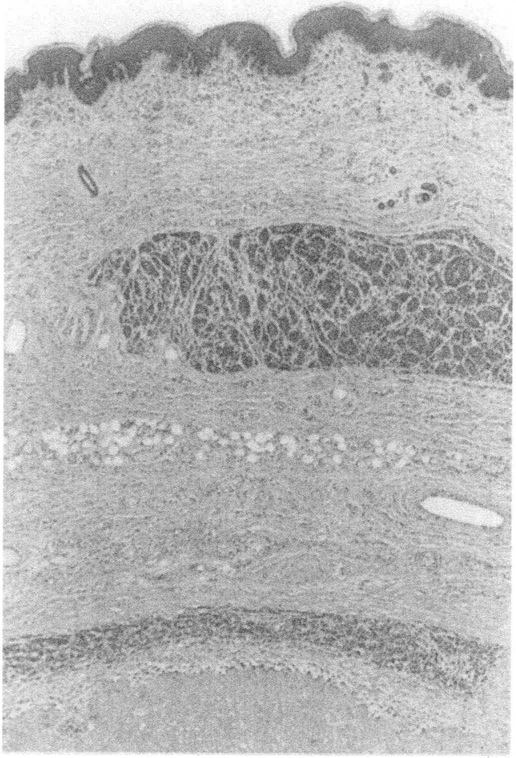

a

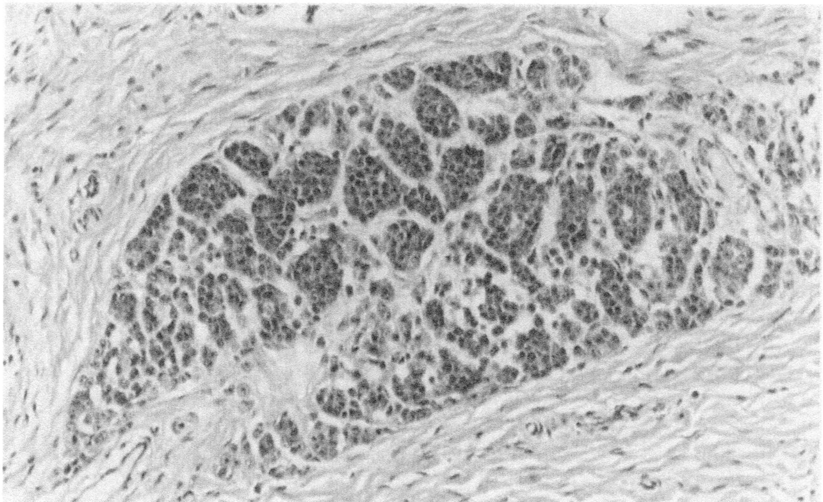

b

Fig. 29a,b. *Malignant melanoma in congenital naevus in an infant.* **a** Nodules of uniform, small atypical melanocytes, with necrosis of the large aggregate at the base of the section, are interspersed with remnants of congenital naevus arranged as small nests in the superficial dermis. **b** Small, solid aggregates of melanoma cells with scanty cytoplasm and hyperchromatic nuclei; inconspicuous, dispersed cells of the congenital naevus in the surrounding fibrillar stroma

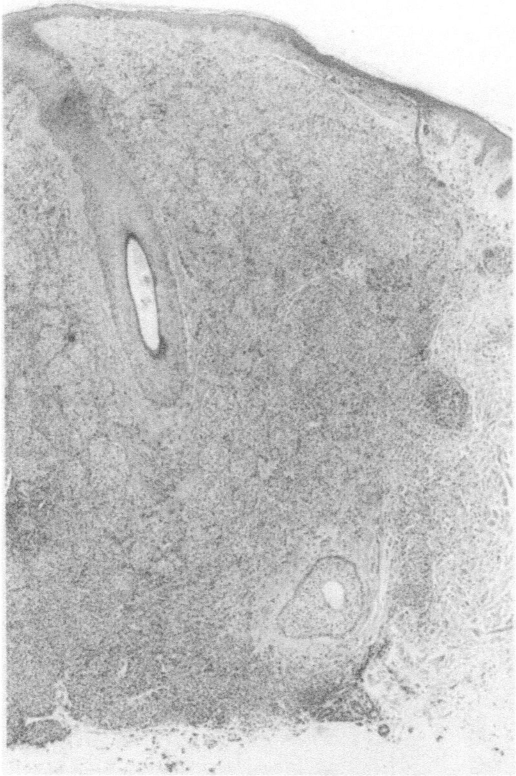

a

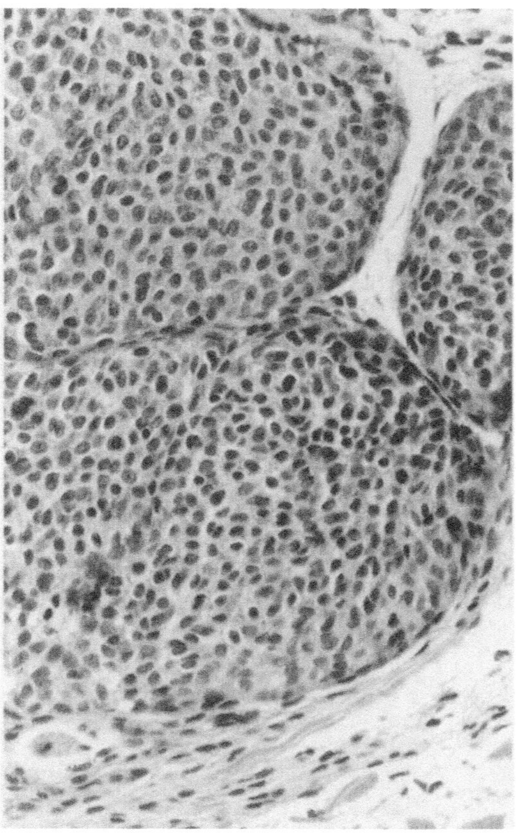

b

Fig. 30a,b. *Minimal deviation melanoma, naevoid cell type.* **a** The invasive component extends into the deep reticular dermis and has an irregular nested pattern. **b** The tumour at the base of the invasive component consists of large groups of relatively small cells with scanty cytoplasm and atypical hyperchromatic nuclei

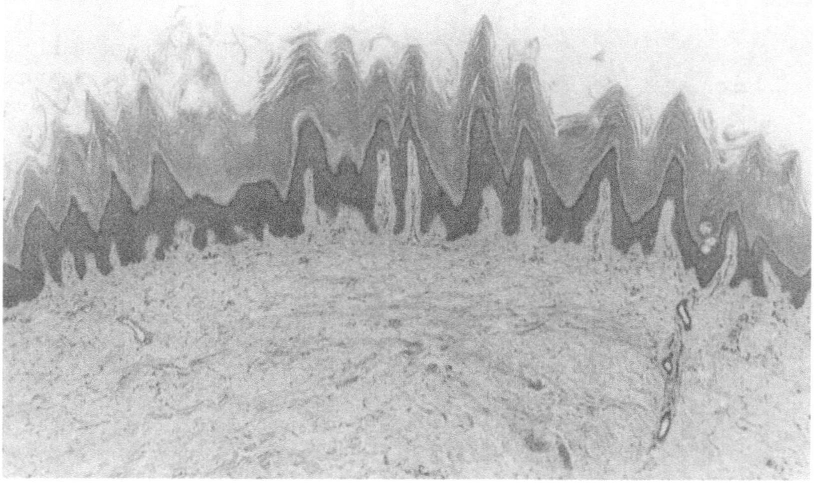

Fig. 31. *Epidermal naevus.* Verrucous epidermal hyperplasia with hyperkeratosis

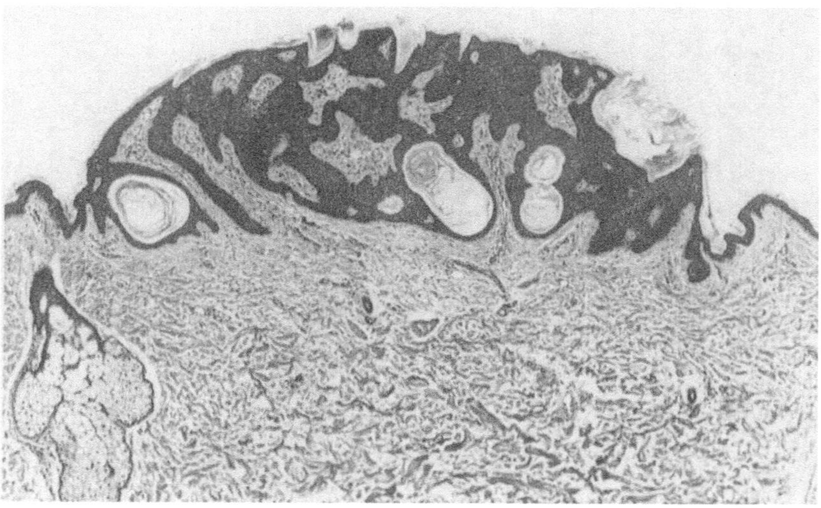

Fig. 32a. *Seborrhoeic keratosis.* Sharply defined, exophytic epidermal tumour with interlocking downgrowths of basaloid cells, papillomatosis and pseudohorn cyst formation

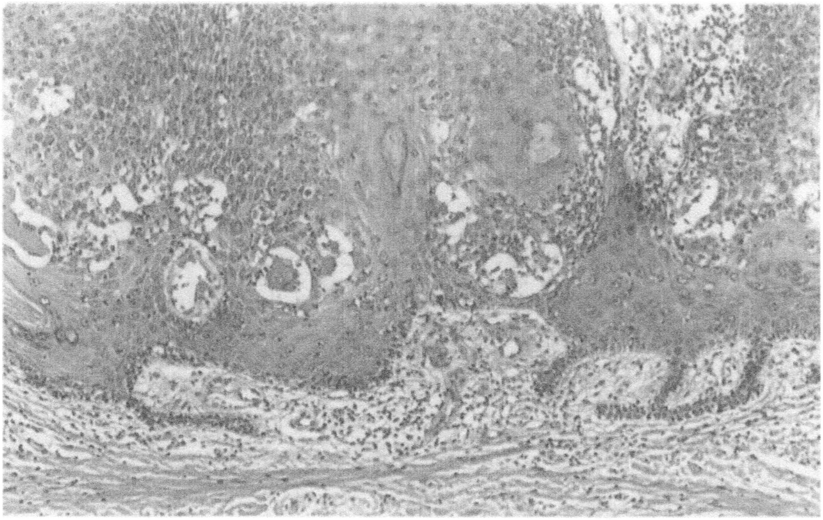

b

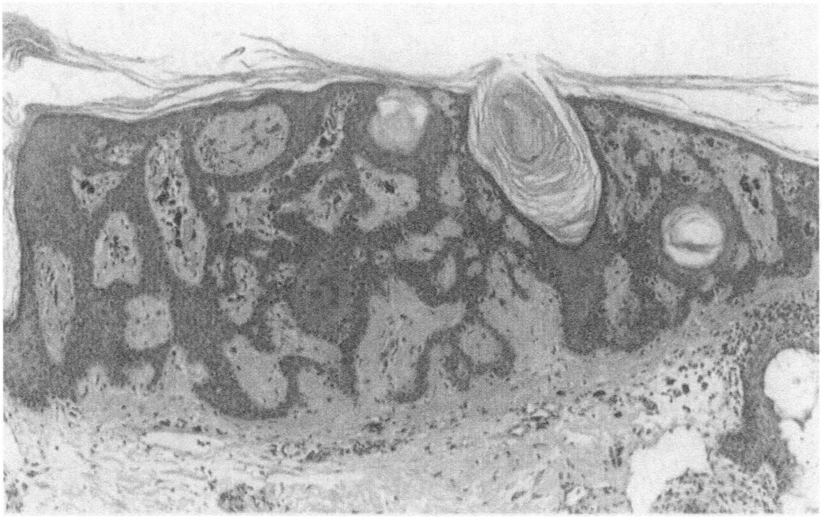

c

Fig. 32b,c. *Seborrhoeic keratosis.* **b** Irritated seborrhoeic keratosis. A patchy infiltrate of lymphocytes in the epithelial tumour with foci of dyskeratosis. **c** Seborrhoeic keratosis, adenoid or reticular pattern

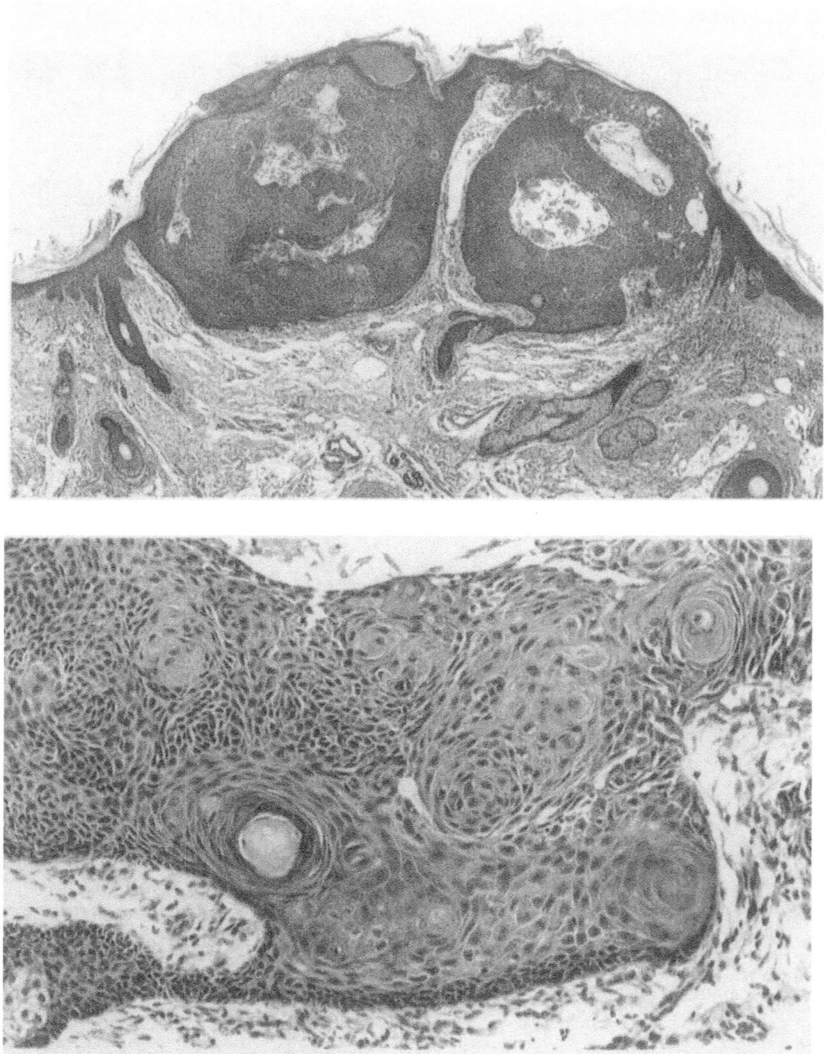

a

b

Fig. 33a,b. *Seborrhoeic keratosis; inverted follicular keratosis variant.* **a** Endophytic, interconnecting downgrowths of squamous epithelium continuous with hair follicles. **b** Epithelial downgrowths including numerous small squamoid eddies

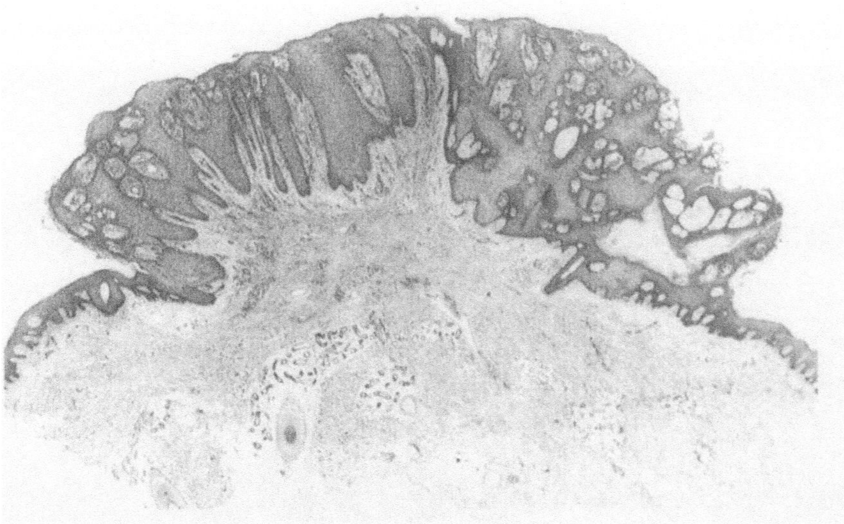

a

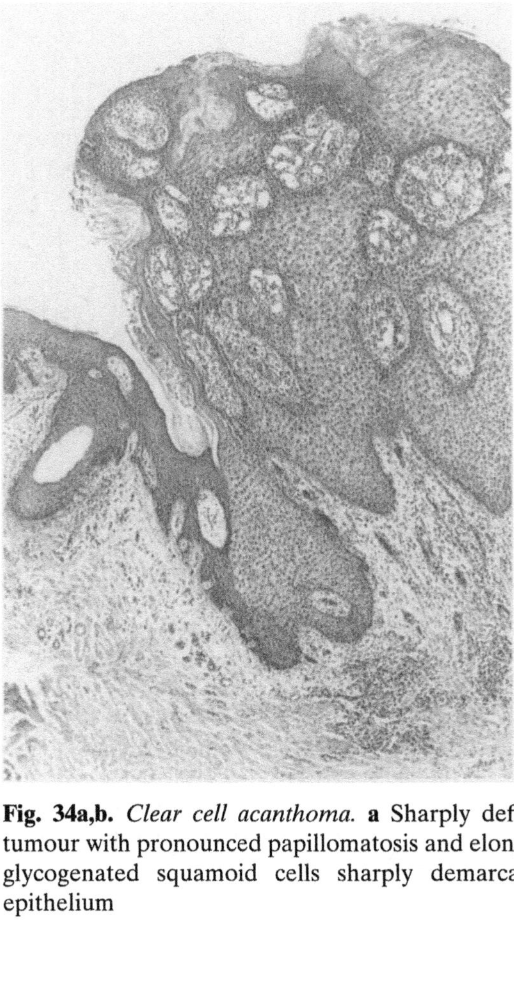

b

Fig. 34a,b. *Clear cell acanthoma.* **a** Sharply defined, protuberant epidermal tumour with pronounced papillomatosis and elongation of rete ridges. **b** Clear, glycogenated squamoid cells sharply demarcated from adjacent normal epithelium

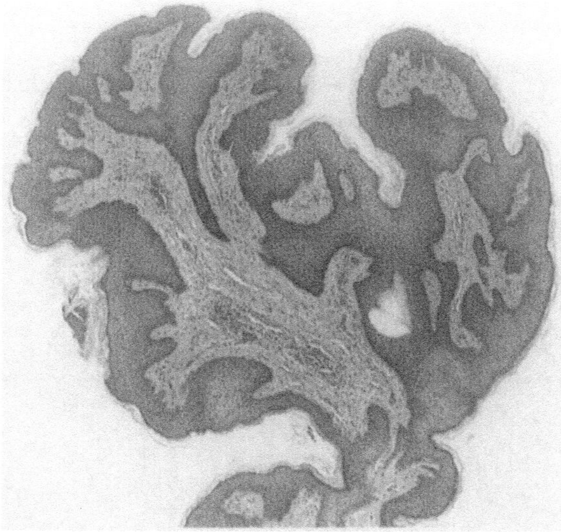

Fig. 35. *Fibroepithelial polyp.* Acanthotic epidermis overlies fibrovascular stroma

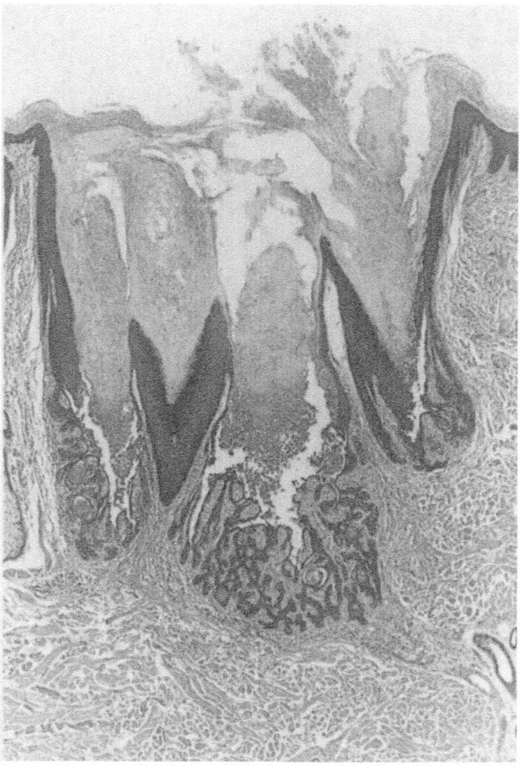

Fig. 36a. *Warty dyskeratoma.* The lesion consists of crater-like downgrowths of squamous epithelium with thick columns of compact keratin overlying suprabasal clefts

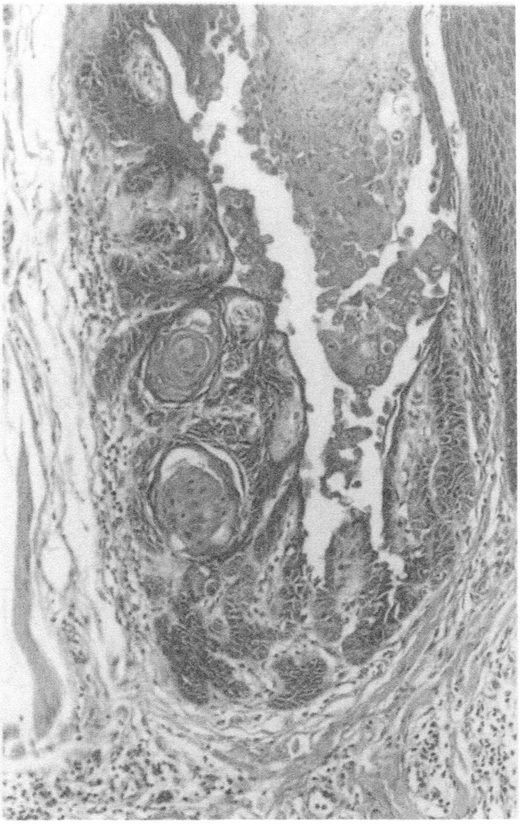

Fig. 36b. *Warty dyskeratoma.* The suprabasal cleft contains acantholytic, dyskeratotic cells overlying villous dermal papillae lined by the retained basal cells

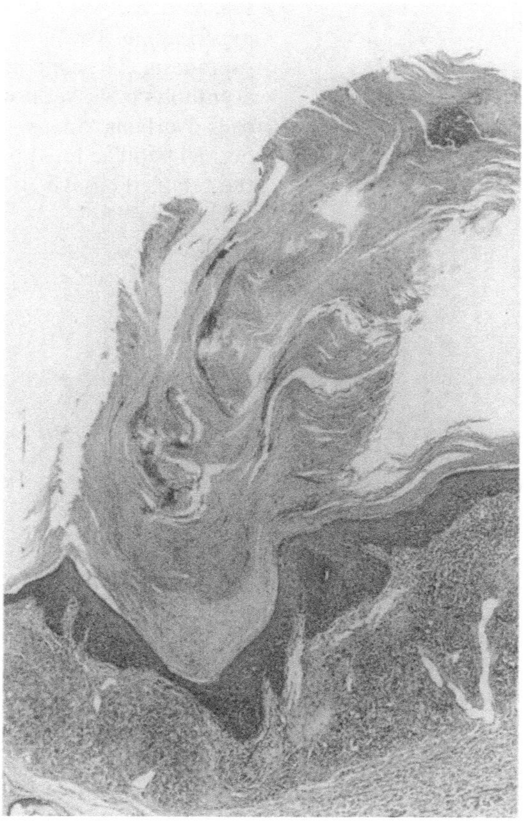

a

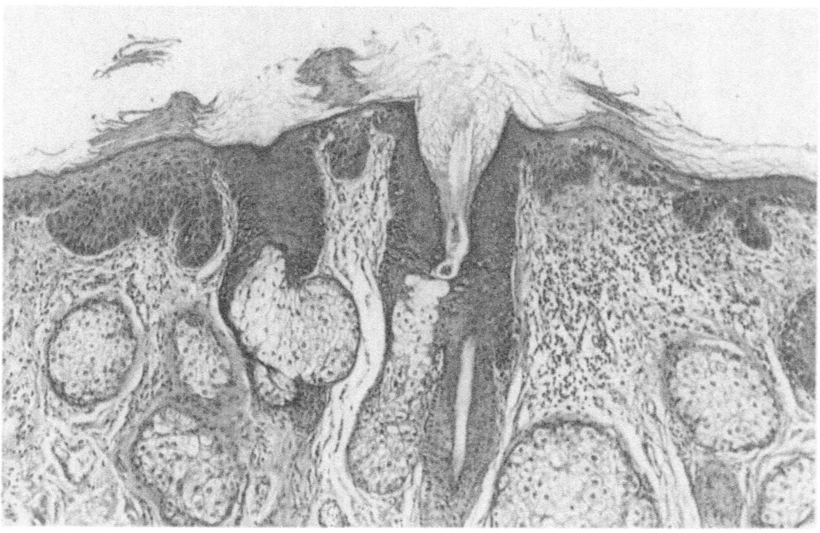

b

Fig. 37a,b. *Actinic keratosis.* **a** A column of parakeratosis overlies acanthotic, atypical squamous epithelium and severe solar elastosis. **b** Several small foci of parakeratosis and moderate squamous cell atypia in blunt downgrowths without invasion of the dermis, in which there is a patchy lymphocytic infiltrate

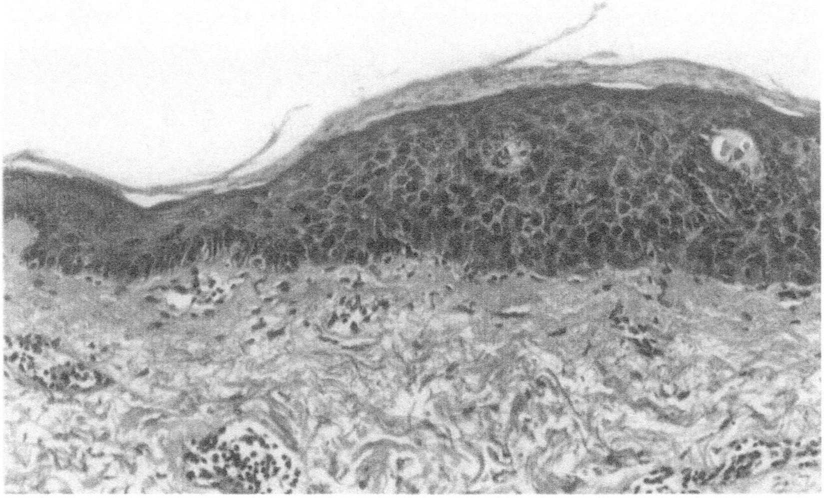

Fig. 38. *Large cell acanthoma.* A sharply defined zone of epidermal thickening in which the keratinocytes have much larger nuclei than those of the adjacent normal epidermis

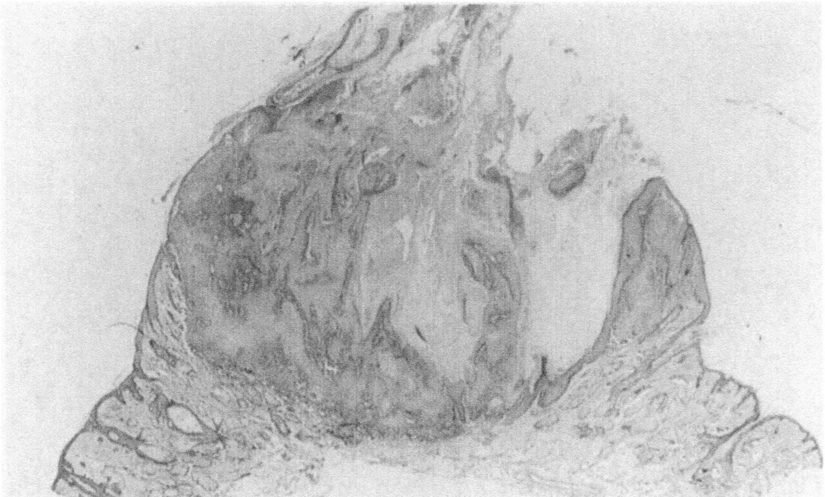

Fig. 39a. *Keratoacanthoma.* The epidermis is raised on either side of a central, irregular, crater-like depression filled with keratotic material, below which there are irregular downgrowths of pale epithelium

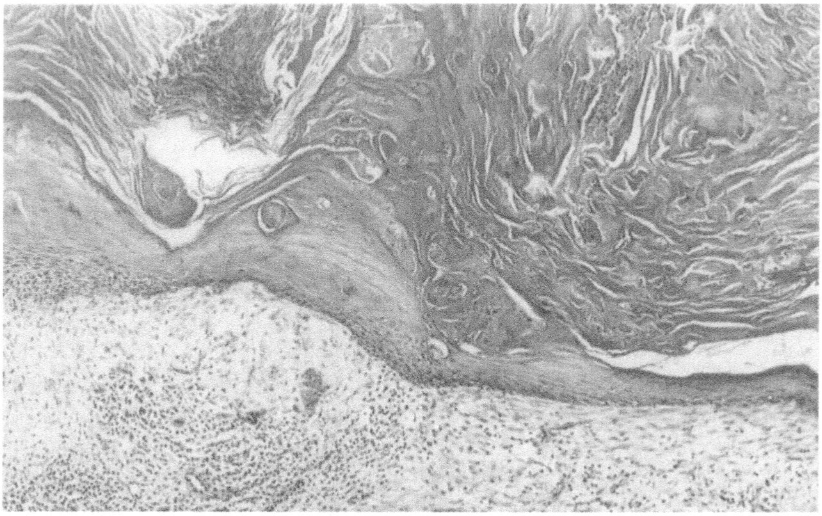

Fig. 39b. *Keratoacanthoma.* The squamous epithelium in the wall of the lesion shows only slight atypia and has a sharp border without dermal invasion

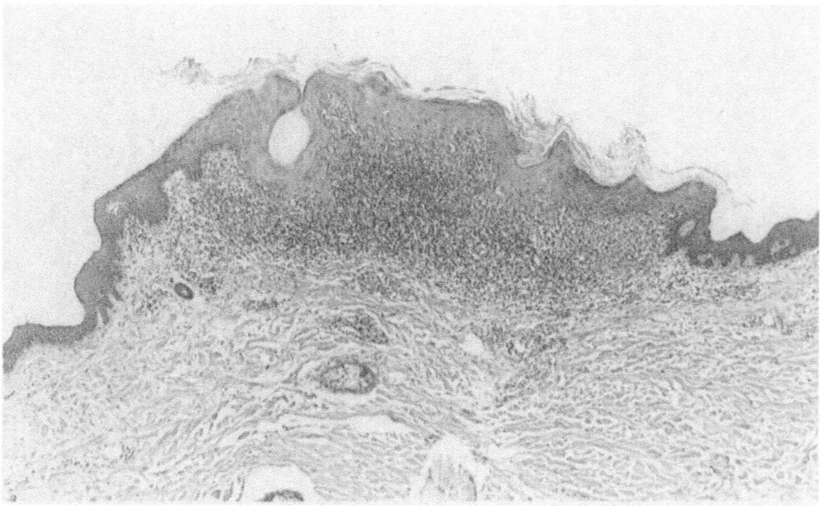

Fig. 40. *Benign lichenoid keratosis (lichen planus-like keratosis).* A band-like lymphocytic infiltrate is applied to the basal layer of the acanthotic epidermis

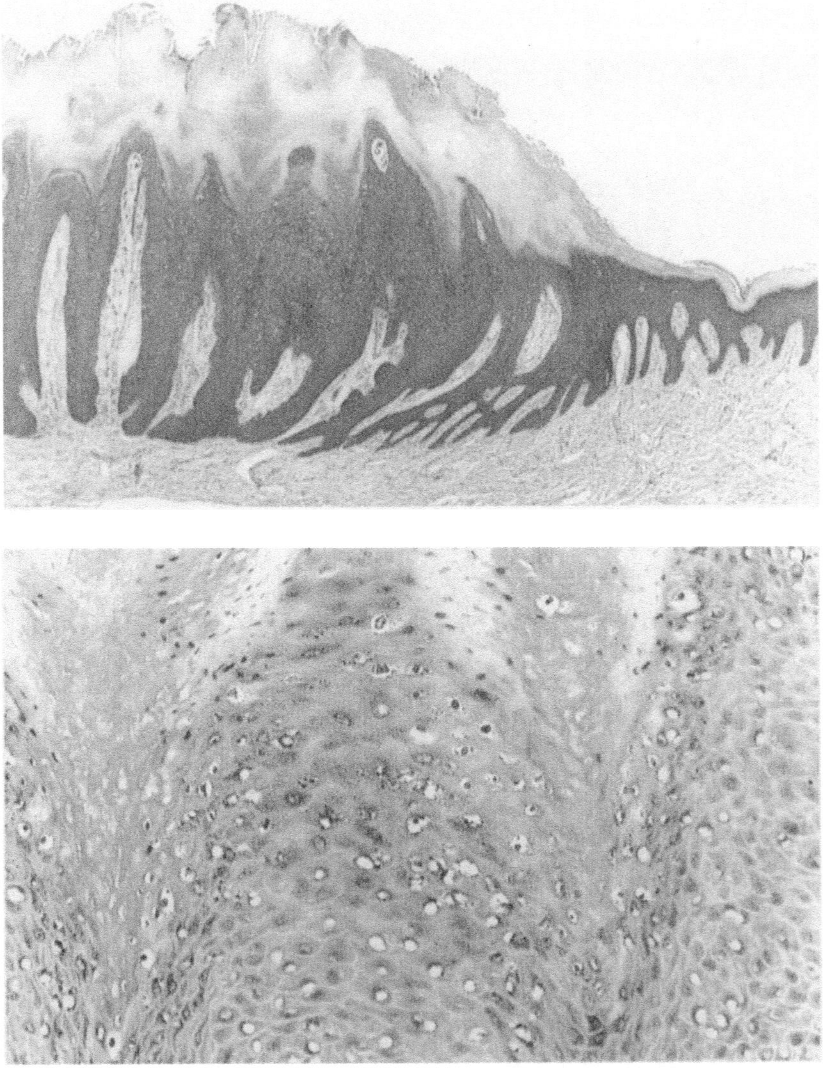

a

b

Fig. 41a,b. *Verruca vulgaris (common wart).* **a** Hyperkeratosis and caps of parakeratosis overlie spires of epidermis with elongated rete ridges slanting inwards towards the centre of the lesion. **b** Parakeratosis overlies keratinocytes with pyknotic nuclei, perinuclear vacuoles and coarse keratohyaline granules

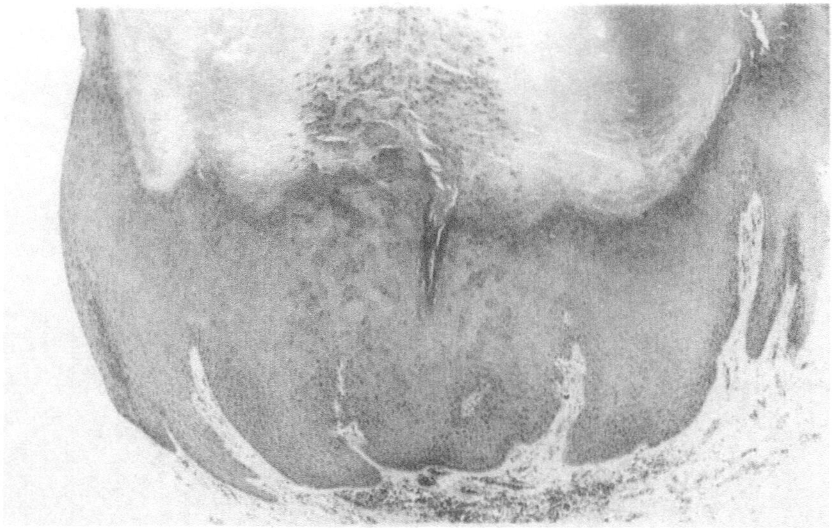

Fig. 42. *Verruca plantaris (plantar wart).* Hyperkeratotic and parakeratotic scale occupies a crater-like depression overlying broad downgrowths of epithelium

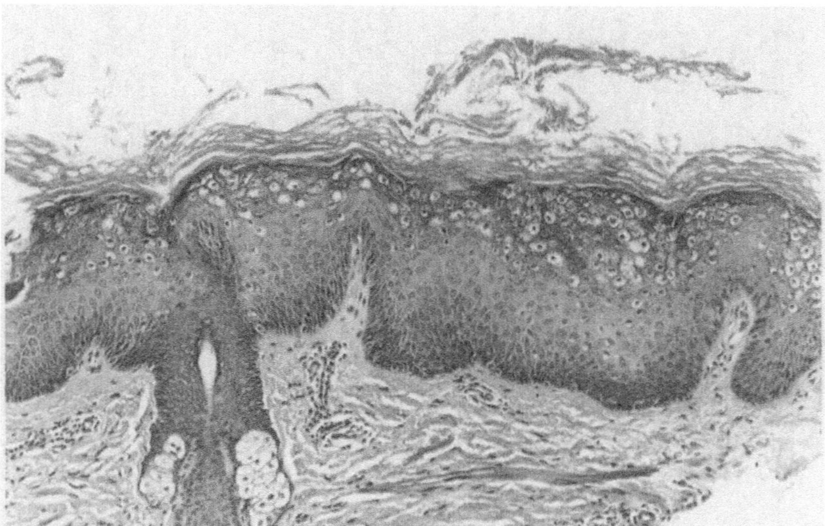

Fig. 43. *Verruca plana (flat wart).* The lesion is flat, with moderate hyperkeratosis, parakeratosis and slight papillomatosis. Numerous koilocytes are present in the upper layers

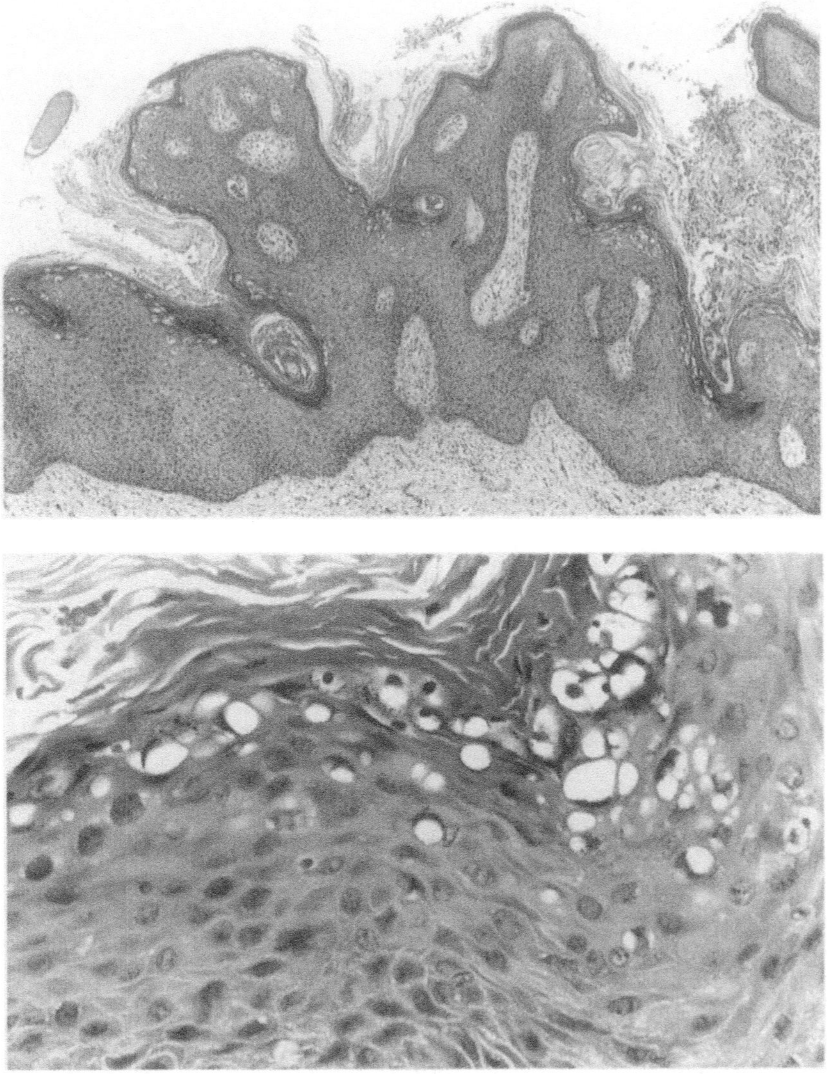

a

b

Fig. 44a,b. *Condyloma acuminatum.* **a** Exophytic and endophytic epithelial hyperplasia. **b** Prominent koilocytes in the upper stratum malpighii

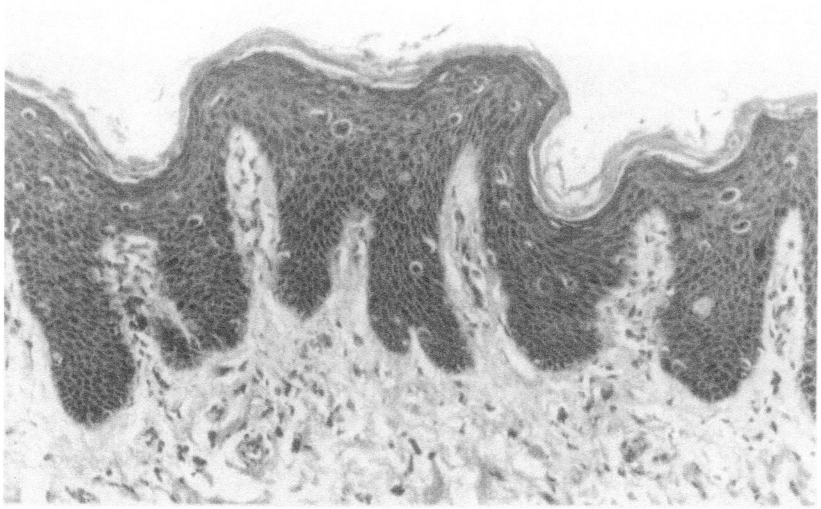

Fig. 45. *Bowenoid papulosis.* Atypical keratinocytes are scattered throughout the epidermis against a background of normal keratinocytes in papillomatous epithelium

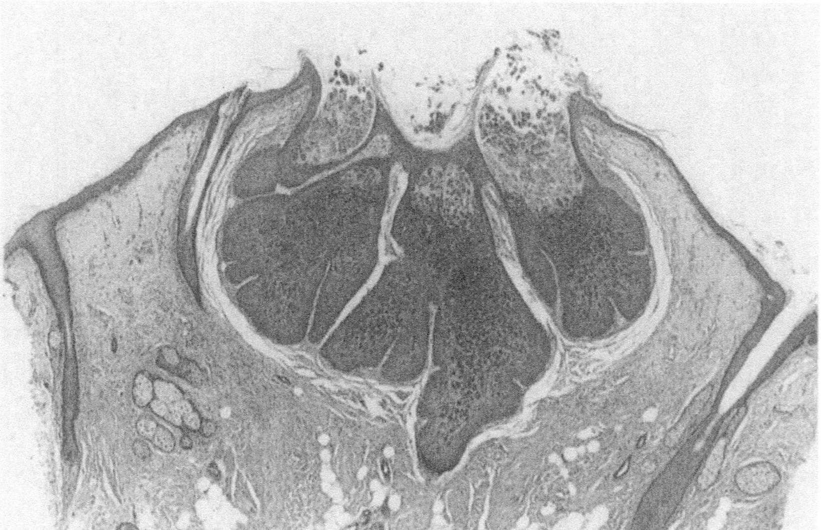

Fig. 46a. *Molluscum contagiosum.* Endophytic, expansile lobules of squamous epithelium

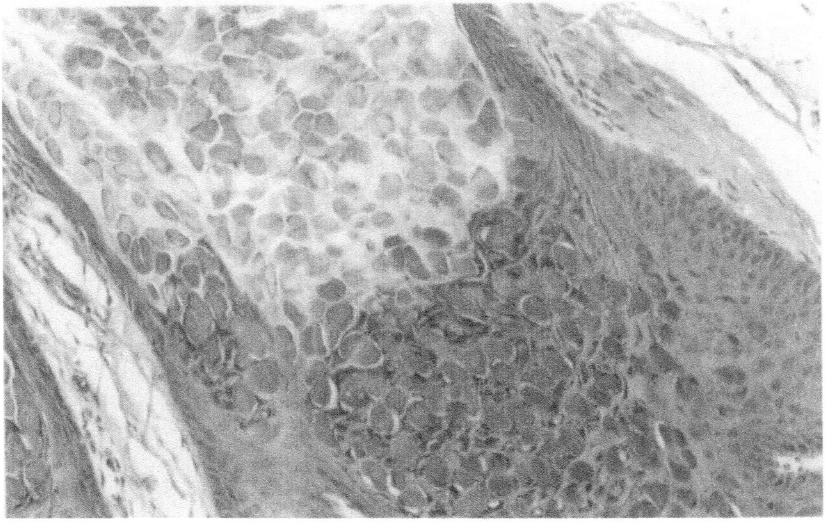

Fig. 46b. *Molluscum contagiosum.* Cytoplasmic inclusion bodies in the upper stratum malpighii and stratum corneum

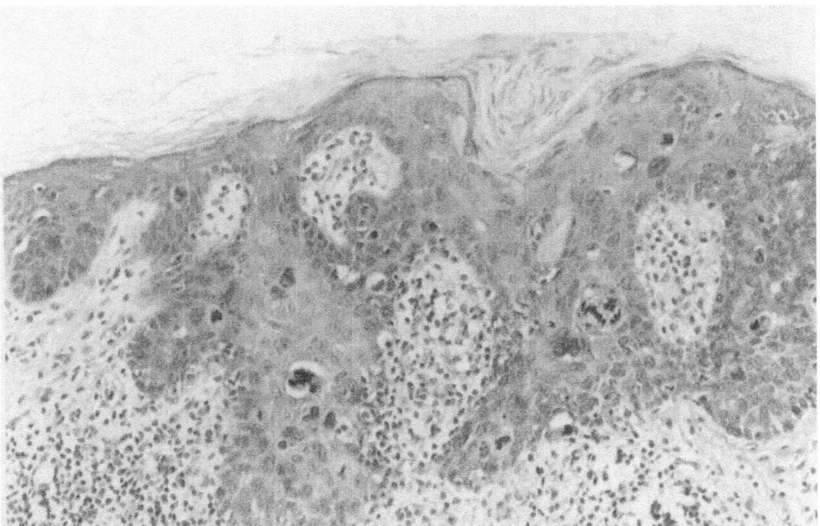

Fig. 47. *In situ squamous cell carcinoma.* Severe squamous cell atypia and distortion of stratification

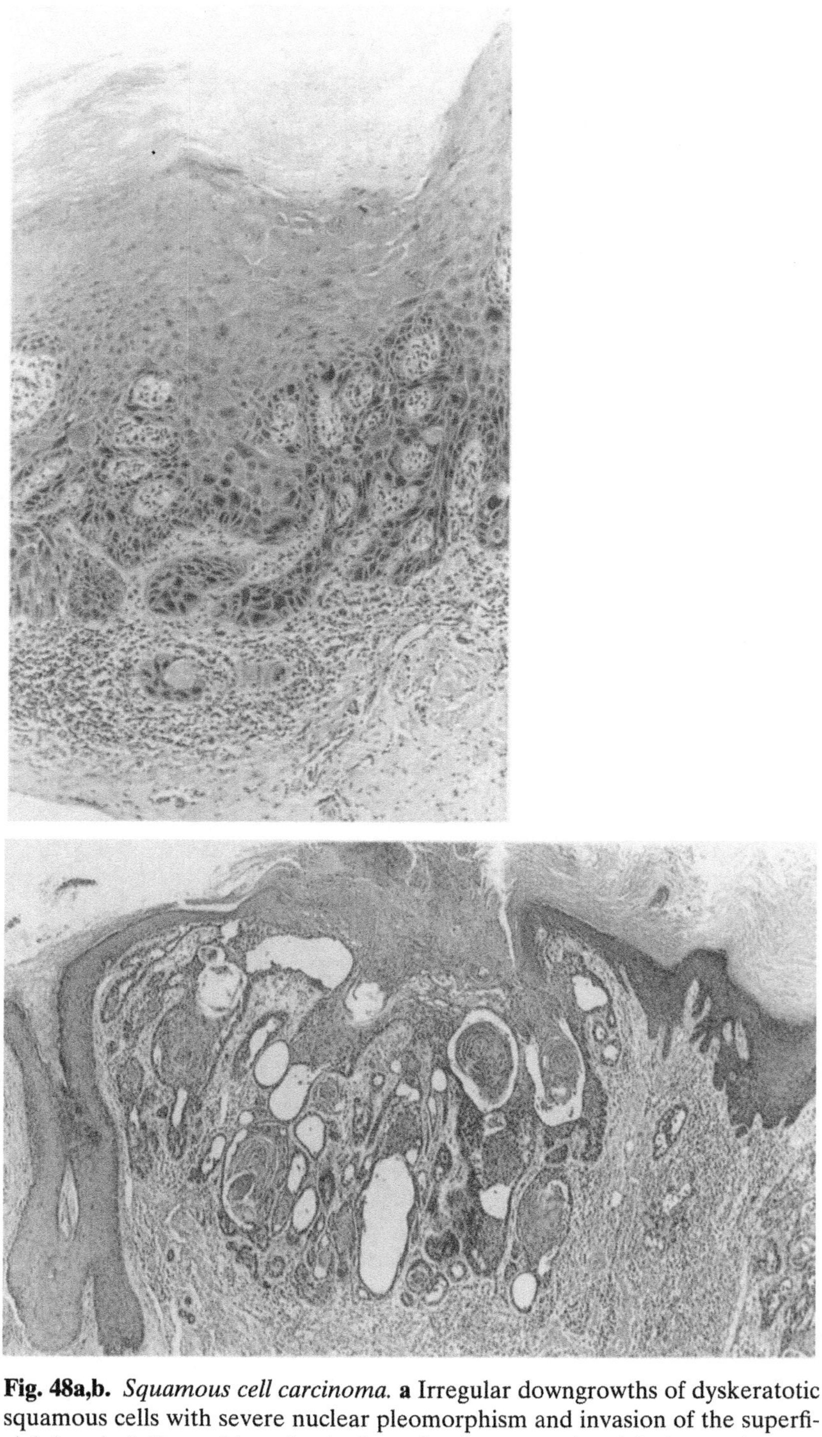

a

b

Fig. 48a,b. *Squamous cell carcinoma.* **a** Irregular downgrowths of dyskeratotic squamous cells with severe nuclear pleomorphism and invasion of the superficial dermis. **b** Dermal invasion by irregular downgrowths of dyskeratotic squamous cells, including cystic or gland-like acantholytic areas

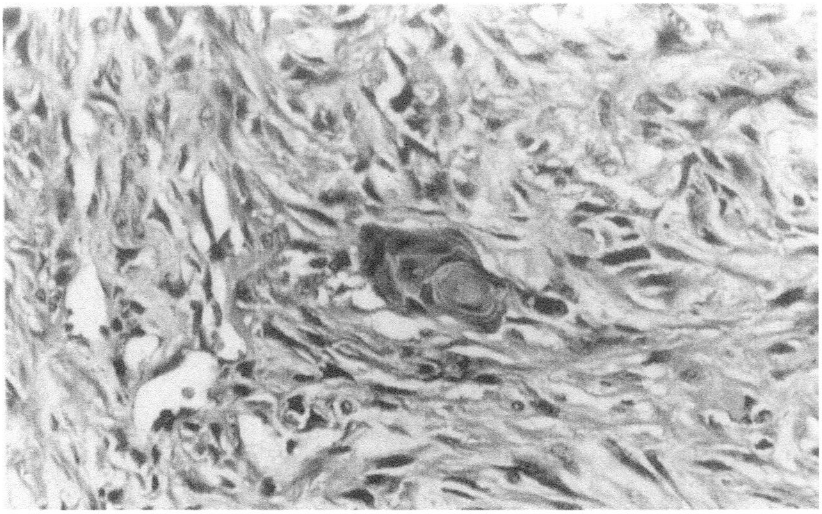

Fig. 49. *Spindle cell squamous cell carcinoma.* A small group of well-differentiated atypical squamous cells surrounded by spindle cells

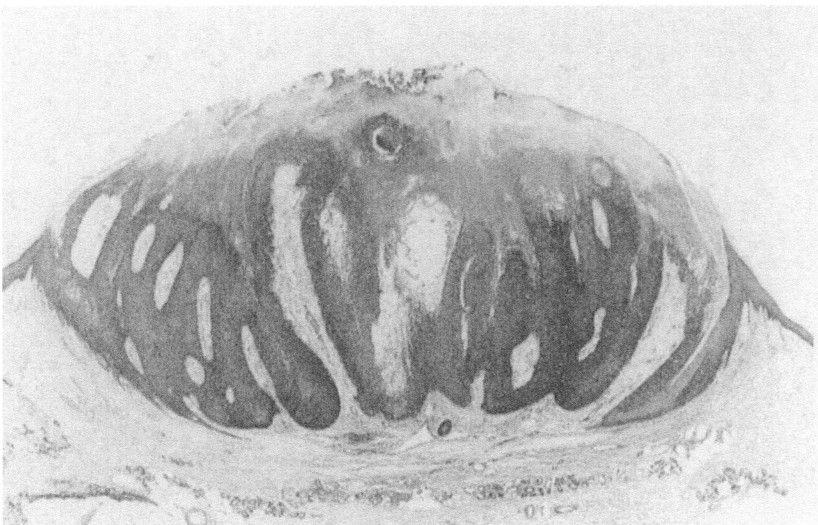

Fig. 50a. *Verrucous squamous cell carcinoma.* Classical verruciform architecture

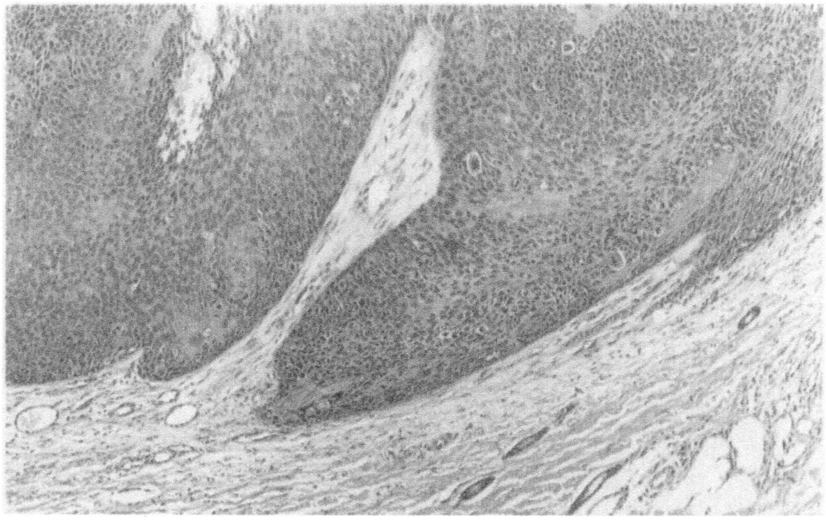

Fig. 50b. *Verrucous squamous cell carcinoma.* Severe squamous cell atypia in the epidermal downgrowths

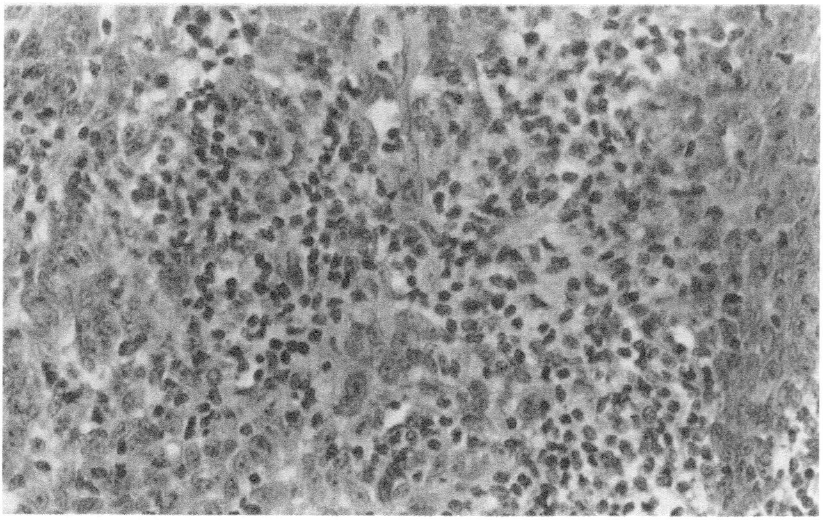

Fig. 51. *Lymphoepithelial squamous cell carcinoma.* Irregular groups of atypical squamous cells separated by a dense infiltrate of lymphocytes

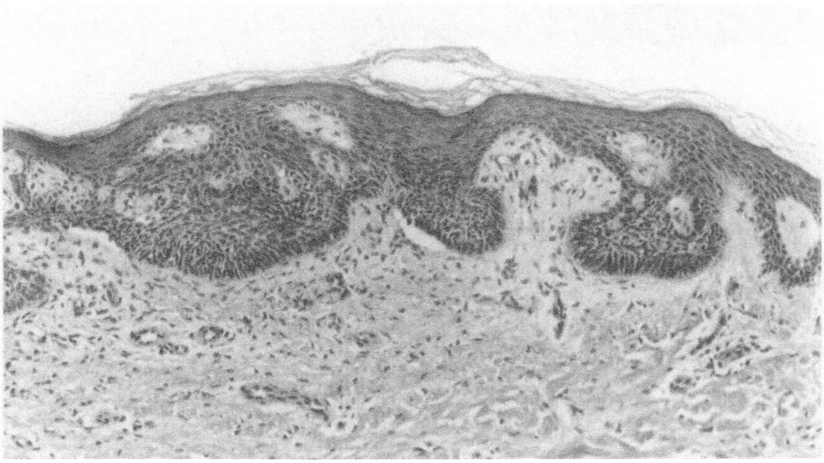

Fig. 52. *Basal cell carcinoma, multifocal superficial type.* Small solid groups of atypical basaloid cells with peripheral palisading push down from the dermo-epidermal junction without invading the dermal stroma

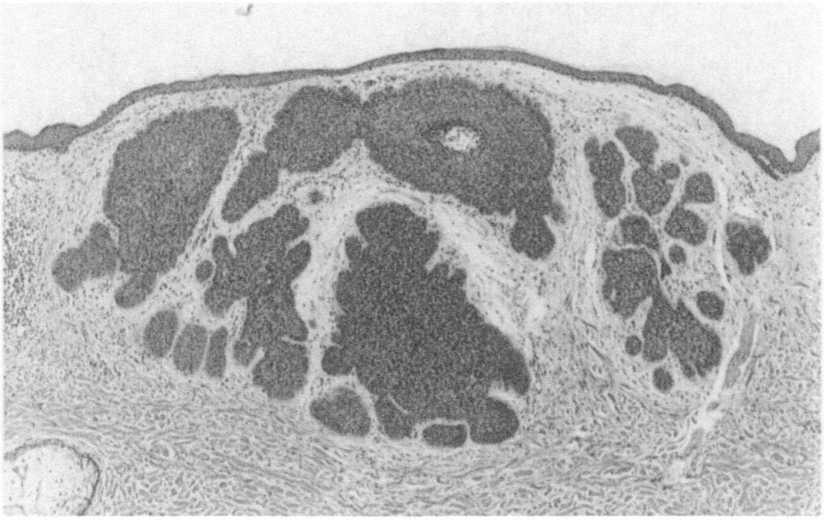

Fig. 53a. *Nodular basal cell carcinoma.* Irregular groups of atypical basaloid cells invade the deep dermis forming a multilobular nodule

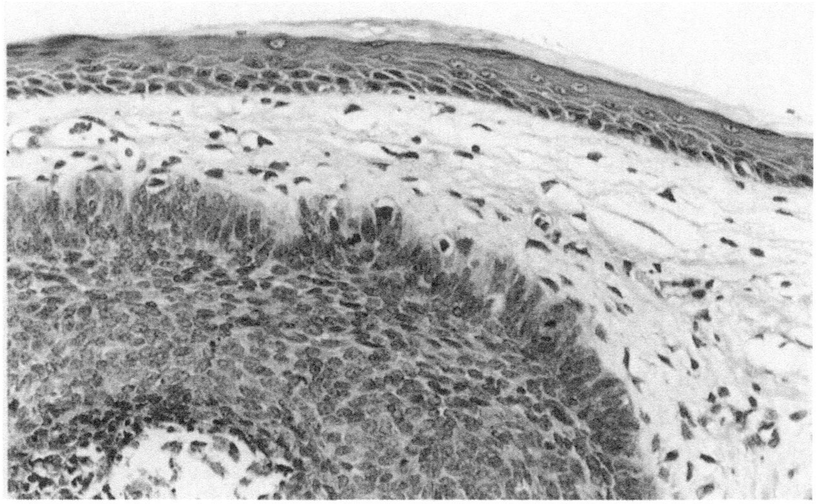

Fig. 53b. *Nodular basal cell carcinoma.* Pronounced peripheral palisading of tumour cells

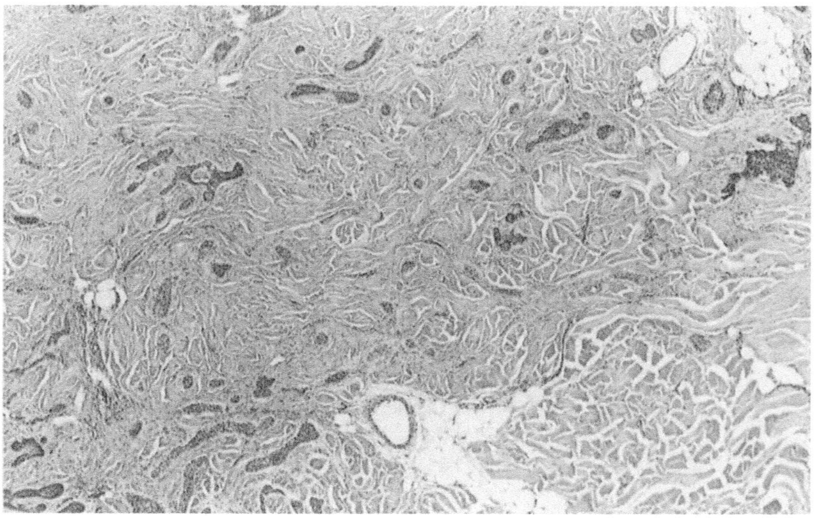

Fig. 54. *Infiltrating, sclerosing (desmoplastic, morpheic) basal cell carcinoma.* Diffuse infiltration of the deep dermis by small solid groups and cords of atypical basaloid cells in a desmoplastic stroma

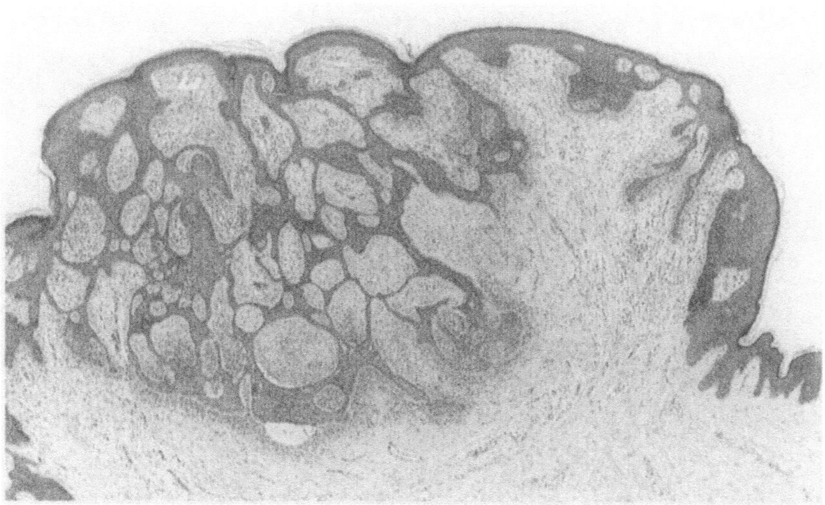

Fig. 55. *Fibroepithelial basal cell carcinoma.* Anastomosing strands of atypical basaloid cells surrounded by cellular stroma

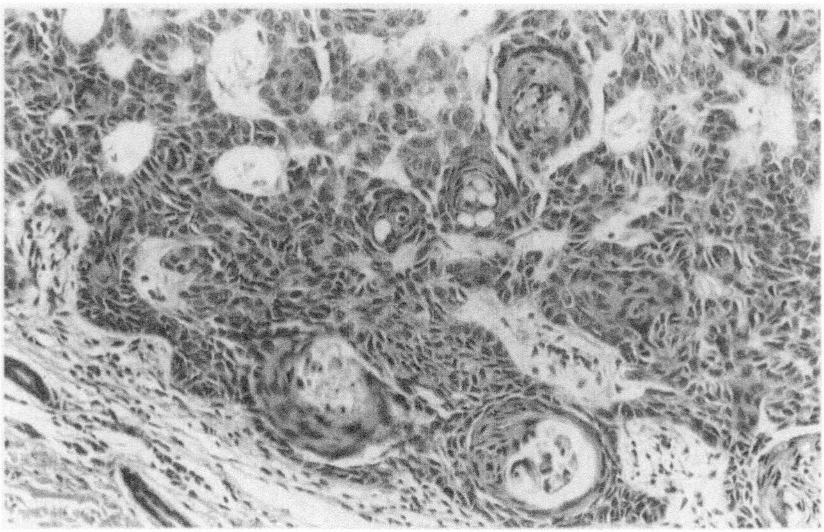

Fig. 56. *Basal cell carcinoma with eccrine differentiation.* Alveolar collections of vacuolated cells and small duct-like structures are present in the centres of tumour nodules

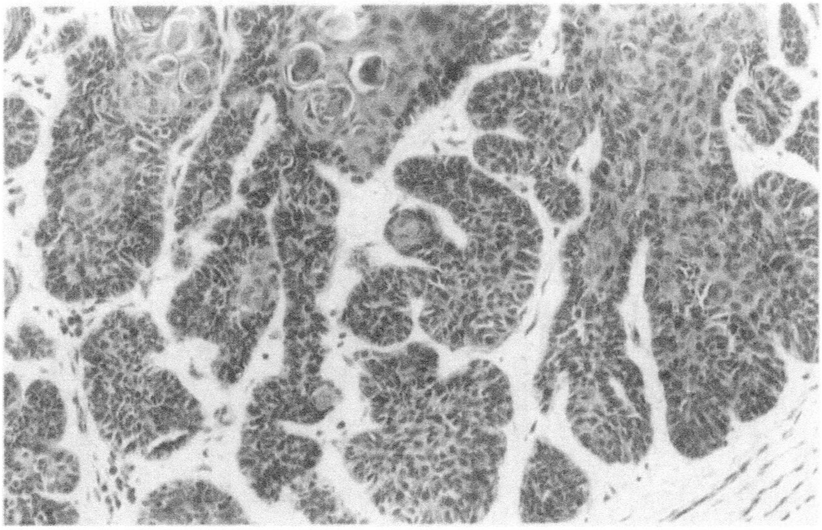

Fig. 57. *Basosquamous carcinoma.* Numerous squamoid eddies and foci of keratinization in irregular groups of otherwise atypical basaloid cells

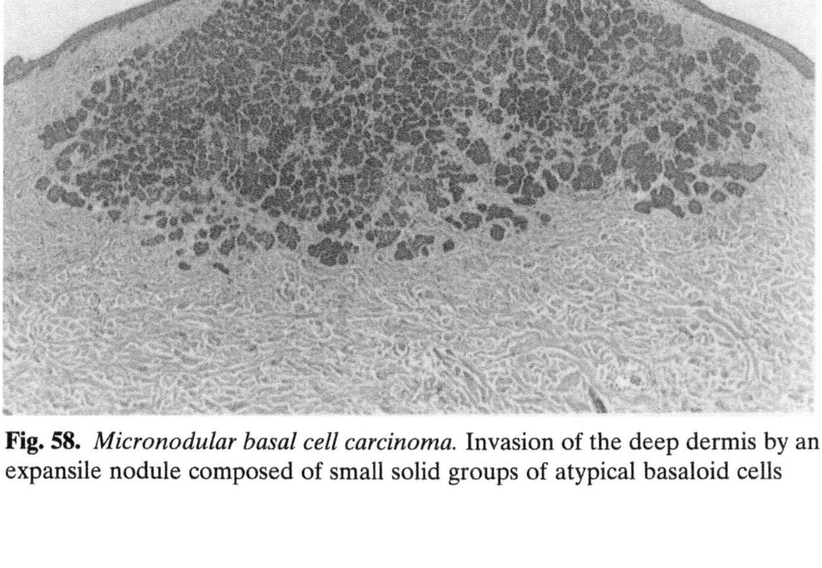

Fig. 58. *Micronodular basal cell carcinoma.* Invasion of the deep dermis by an expansile nodule composed of small solid groups of atypical basaloid cells

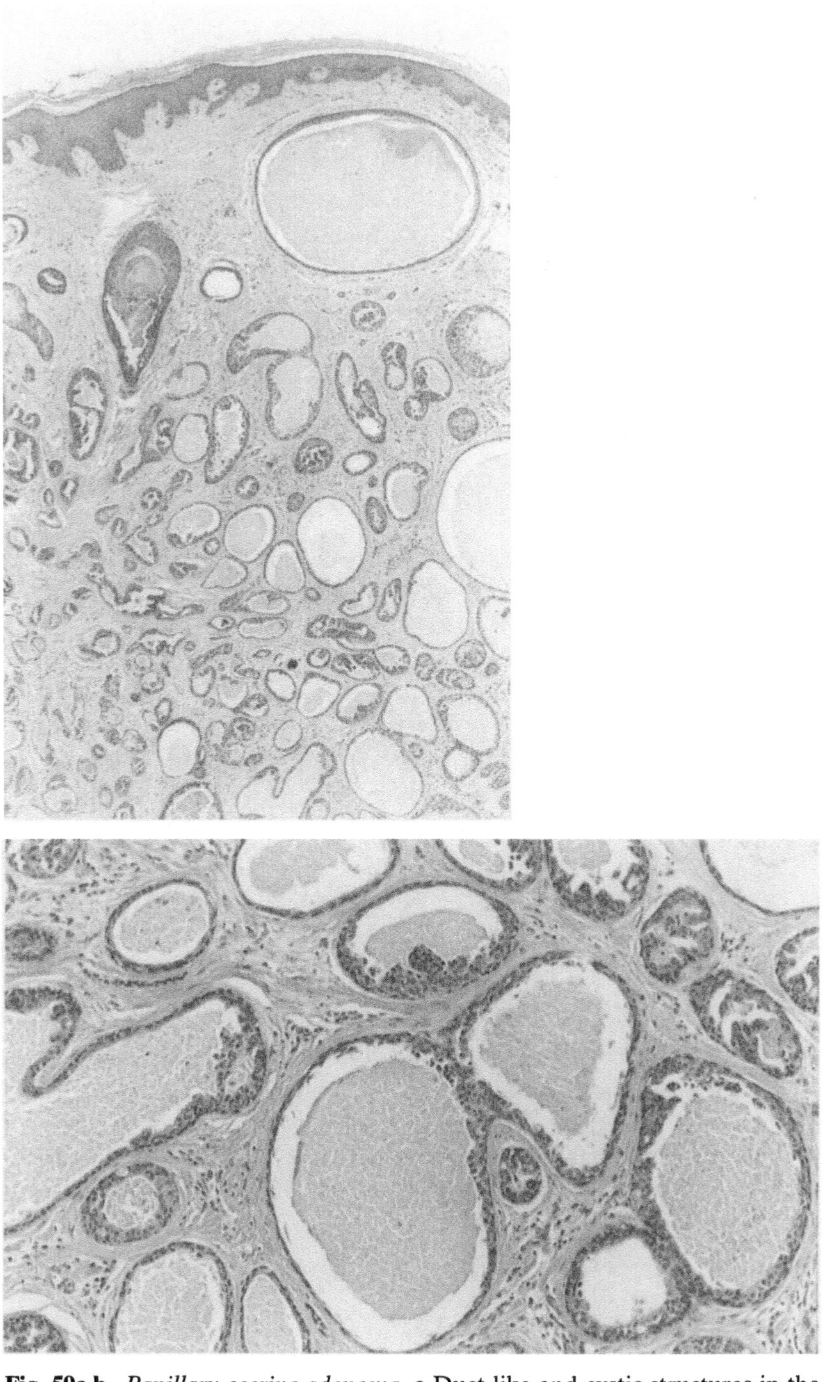

Fig. 59a,b. *Papillary eccrine adenoma.* **a** Duct-like and cystic structures in the superficial and deep dermis. **b** The more dilated structures are lined by cuboidal and cuticular epithelium. Small papillary projections into the lumen are more plentiful in the smaller ductal structures

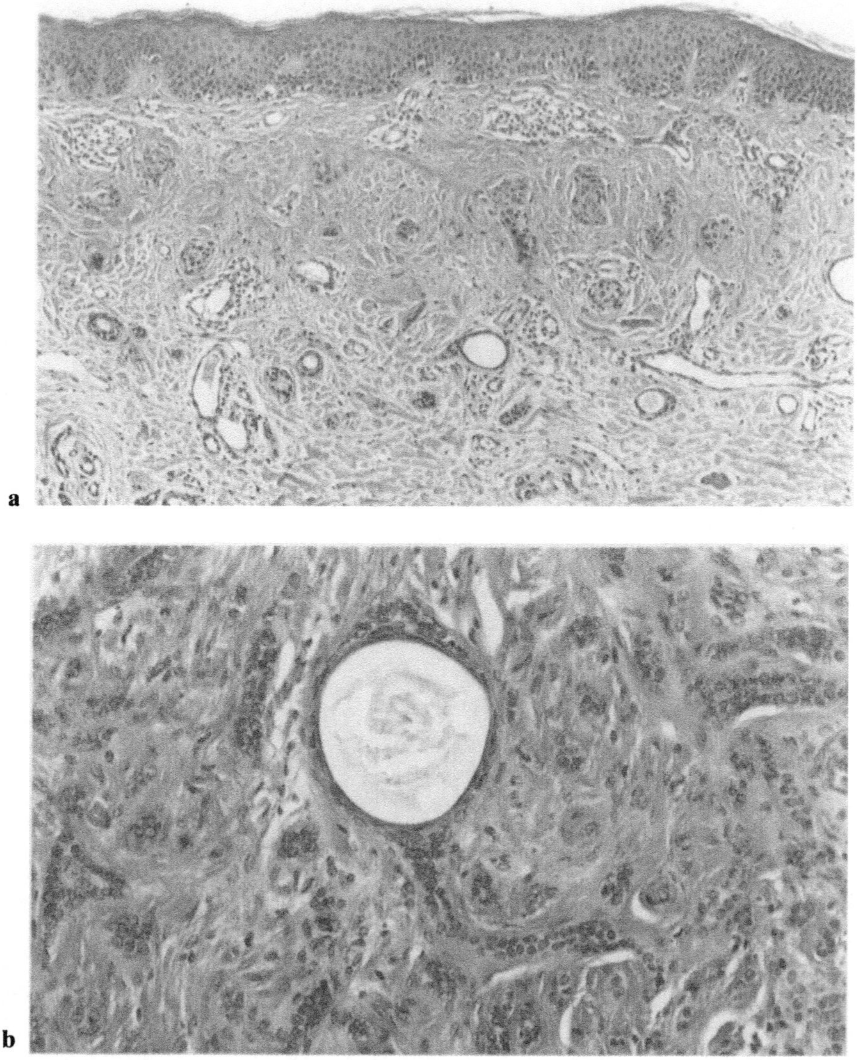

Fig. 60a,b. *Syringoma.* **a** Small solid groups and strands of uniform cuboidal epithelium and ductal structures are embedded in a collagenous stroma. **b** Typical comma or tadpole-like shape of a ductal structure lined by flattened cuticular epithelium with an attached tail, i.e. a solid cord of cuboidal epithelium

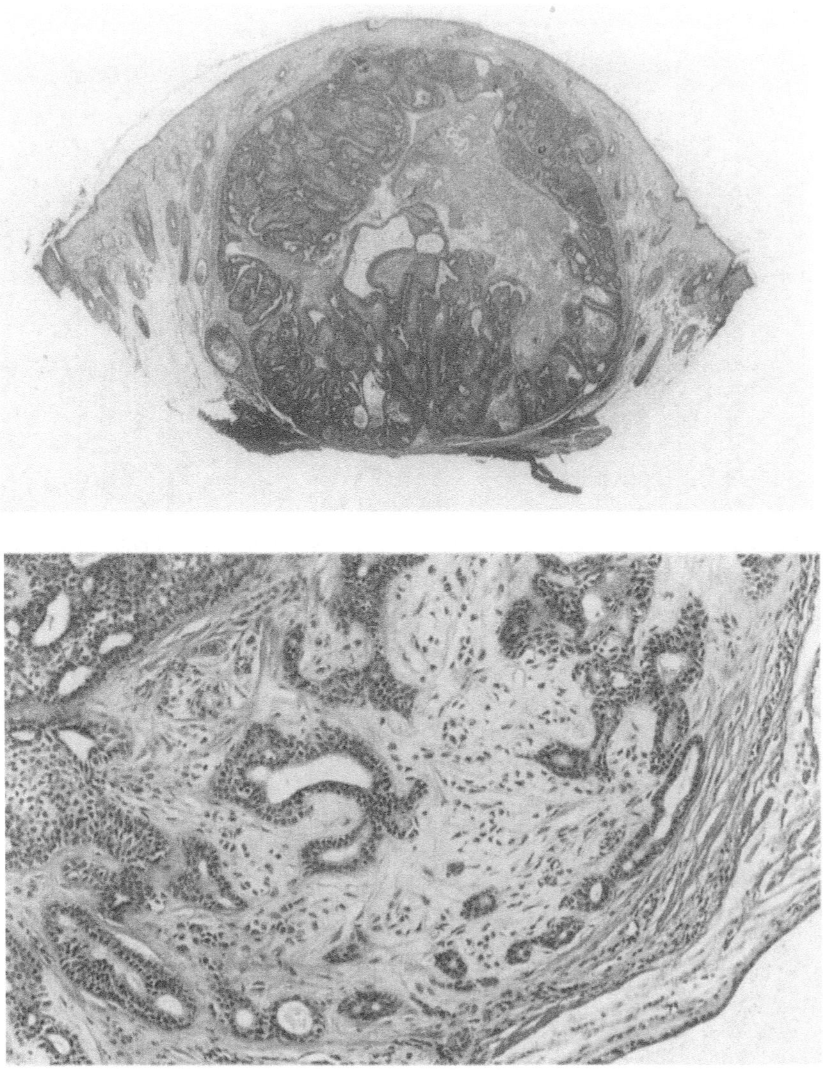

a

b

Fig. 61a,b. *Mixed tumour of skin (chondroid syringoma).* **a** A circumscribed nodular tumour in the dermis and subcutis including solid and cystic areas. **b** Ductal structures lined by cuboidal epithelium embedded in chondroid stroma containing spindle cells

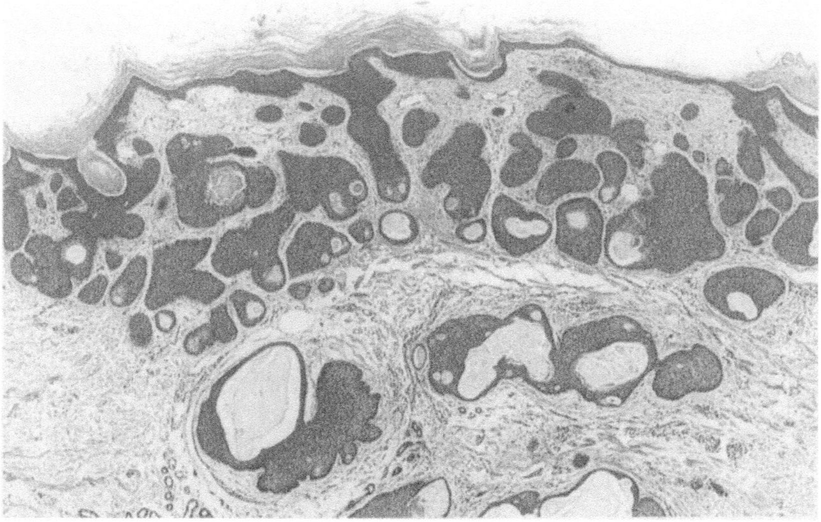

Fig. 62. *Eccrine poroma.* Groups of uniform, small squamoid cells in the epidermis and within the dermis, some containing ductal structures

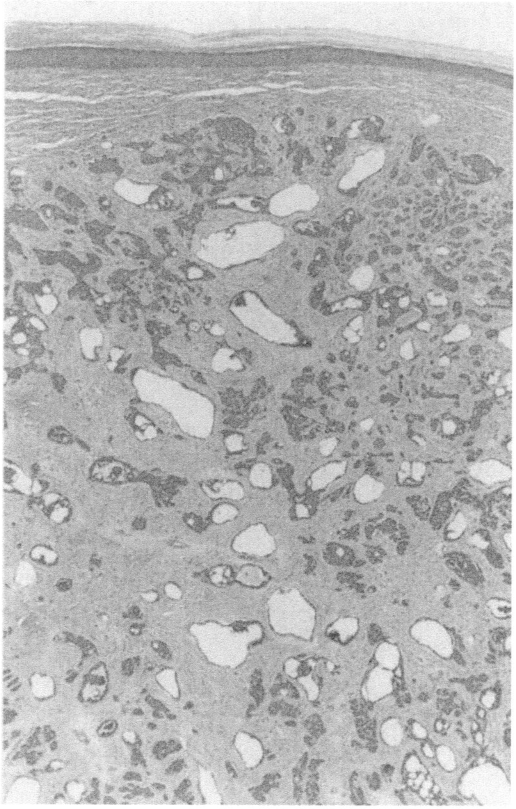

Fig. 63a. *Dermal duct tumour.* Entirely intradermal poroma-like tumour composed of solid aggregates of small squamoid cells and ductal structures

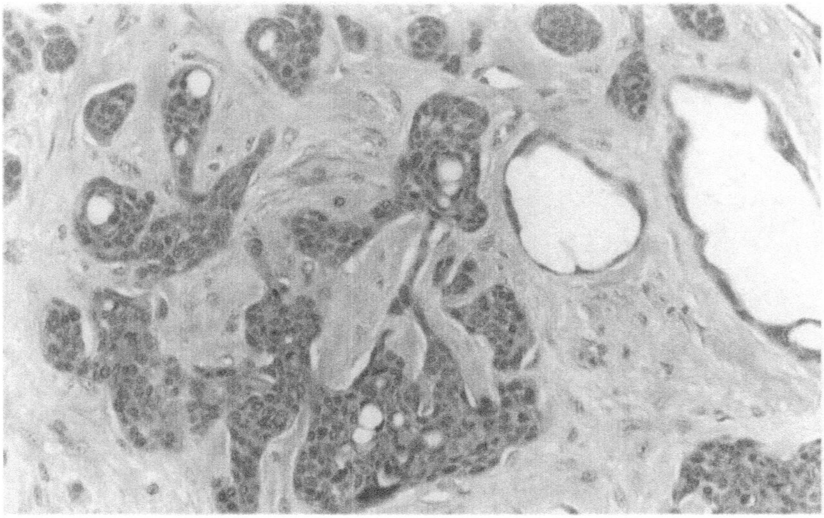

Fig. 63b. *Dermal duct tumour.* Thin-walled cystic structures and smaller lumina in more cellular tumour islands

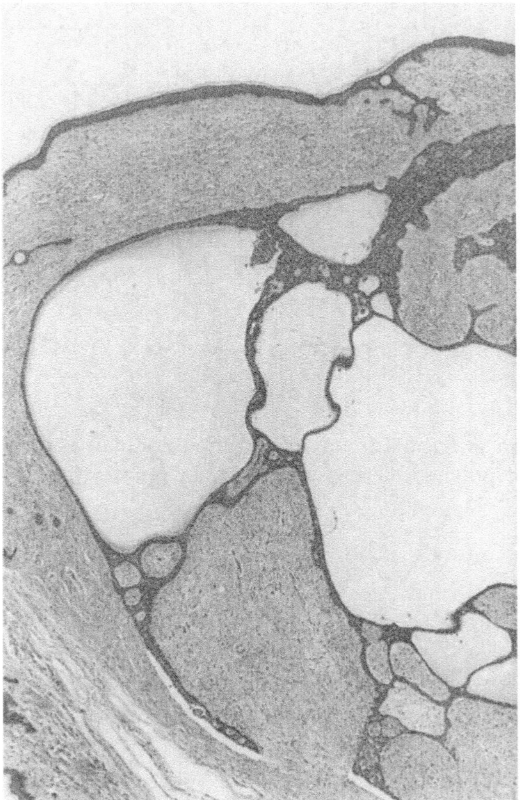

Fig. 64. *Syringofibro-adenoma.* Anastomosing cords of cuboidal epithelium surround vascular fibrous stroma and cystic areas

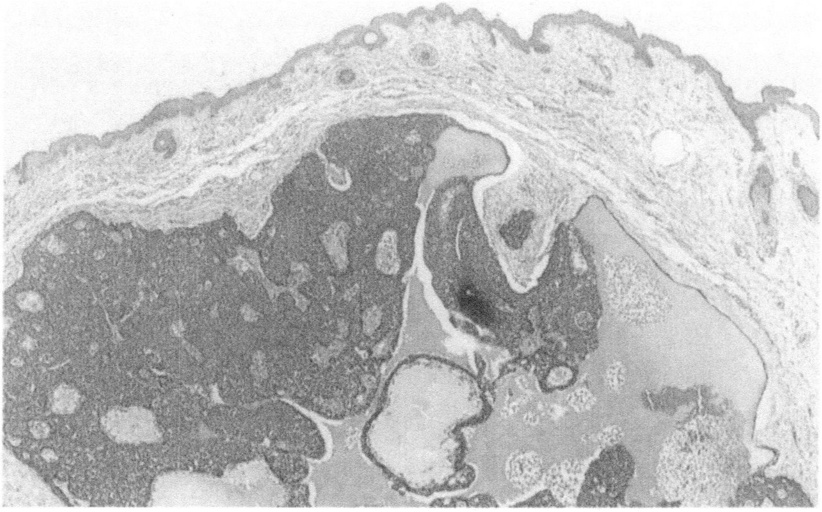

a

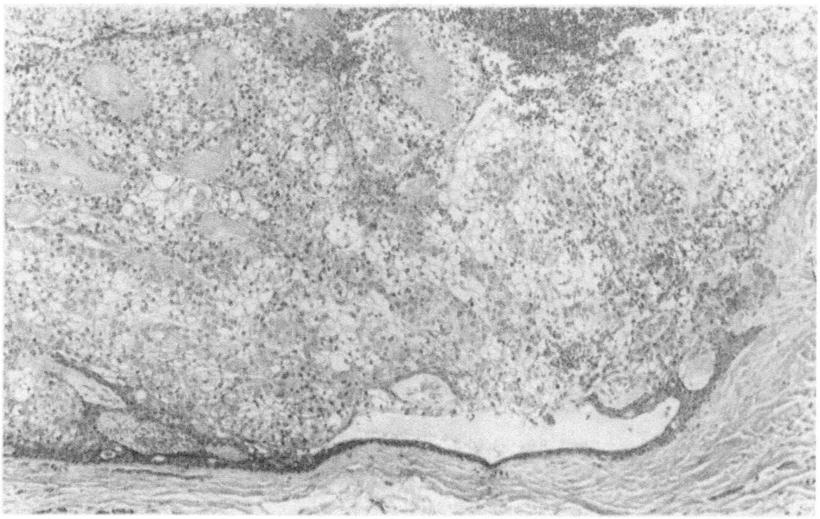

b

Fig. 65a,b. *Nodular hidradenoma.* **a** Circumscribed, multilobular, solid and cystic tumour. **b** Sheets of polyhedral cells with clear cytoplasm (clear cell hidradenoma)

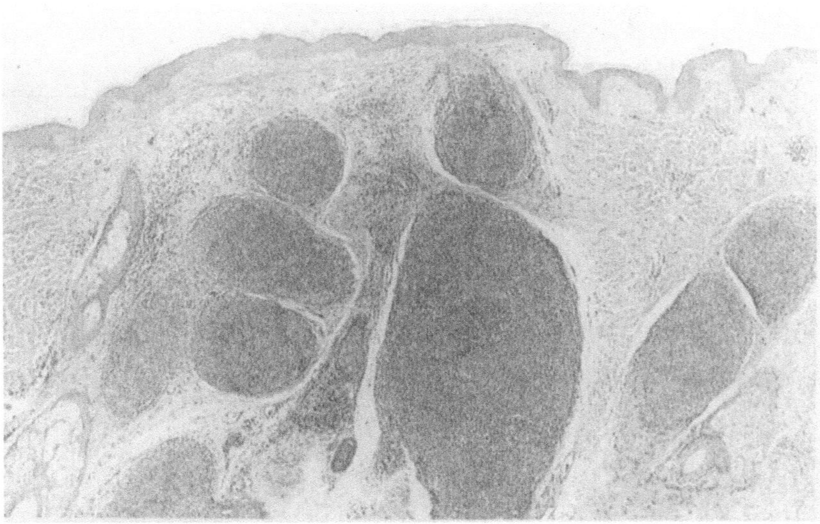

a

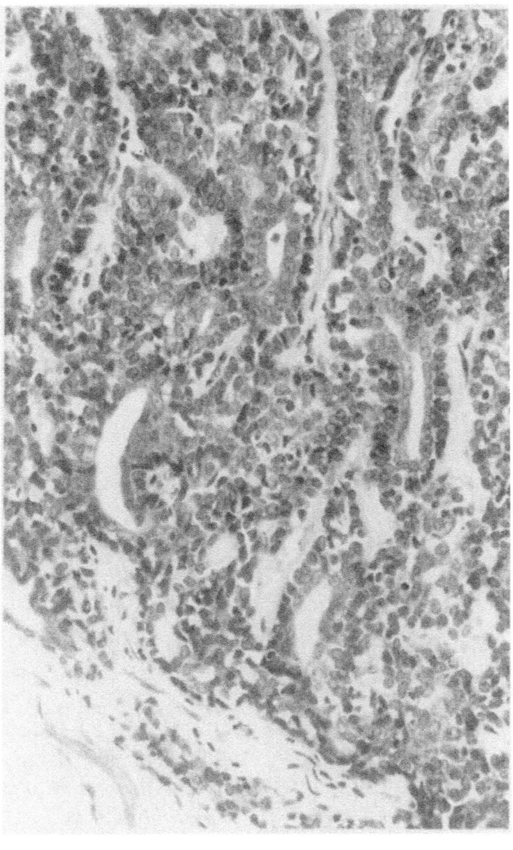

b

Fig. 66a,b. *Eccrine spiradenoma.* **a** Circumscribed densely cellular nodules in the dermis. **b** The nodules are composed of cuboidal cells with dark nuclei, cuboidal cells with pale nuclei, and lymphocytes

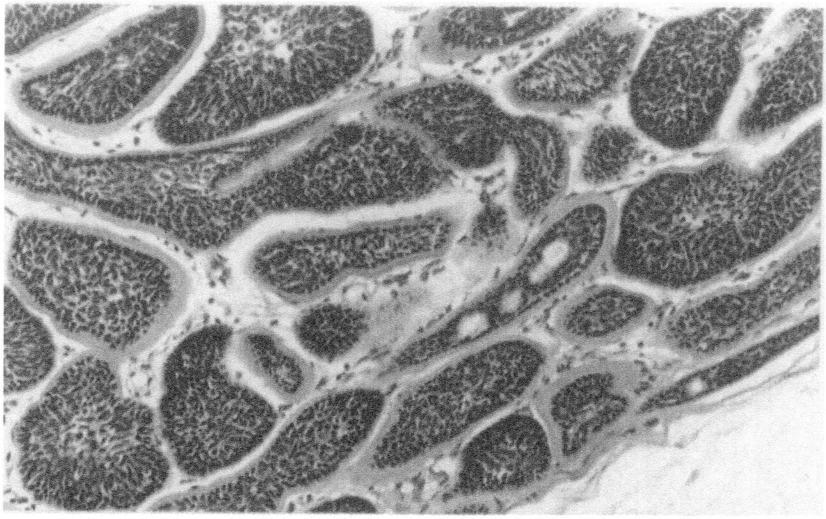

Fig. 67. *Cylindroma.* Hyaline bands surround peripheral layers of basaloid cells and central paler cells; small ductal structures are lined by cuboidal cells

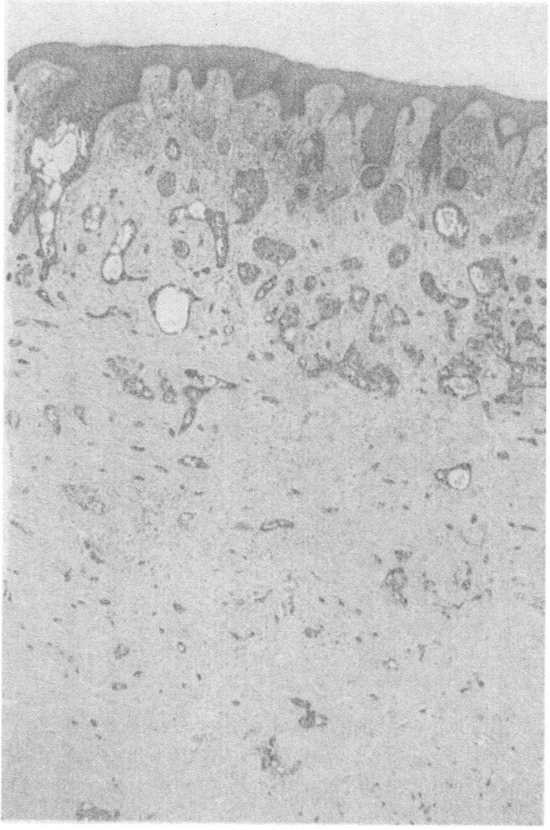

Fig. 68a. *Sclerosing sweat duct carcinoma (syringomatous carcinoma).* Diffuse invasion by small groups of cells embedded in a sclerotic stroma

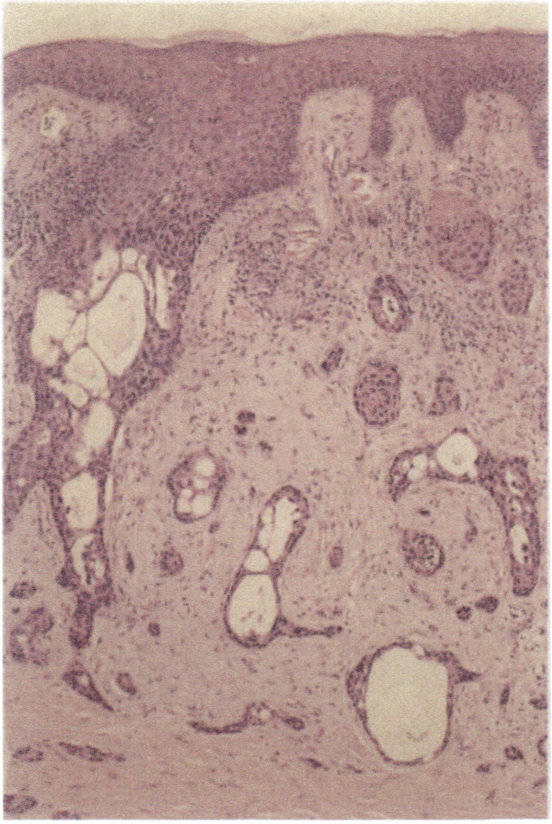

Fig. 68b. *Sclerosing sweat duct carcinoma (syringomatous carcinoma)*. Solid groups of cuboidal cells, small ductal structures and larger, thin-walled cysts are present in the superficial layers. This tumour involves an acrosyringium

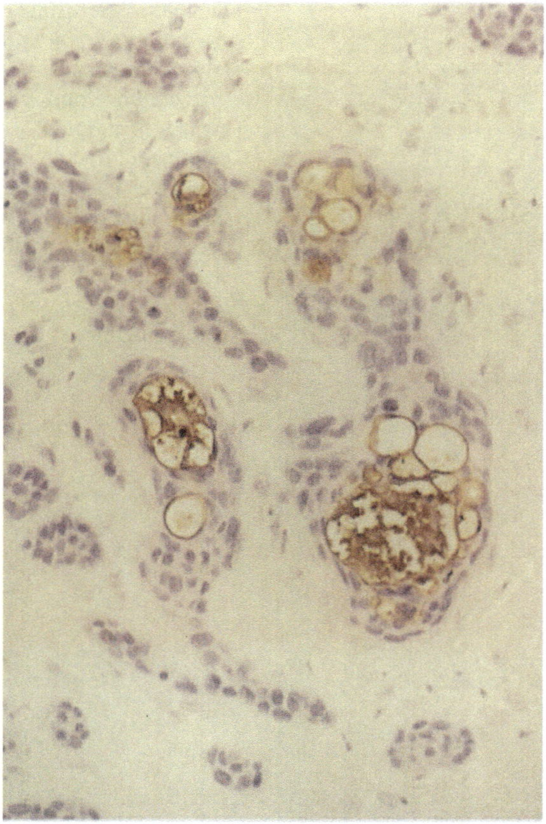

Fig. 68c. *Sclerosing sweat duct carcinoma (syringomatous carcinoma).* Positive immunostaining for carcino-embryonic antigen in the ductal and alveolar structures

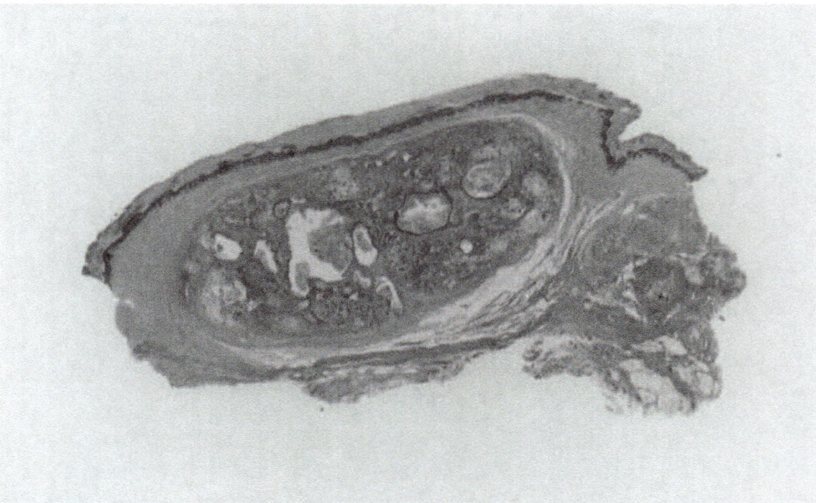

Fig. 69a. *Malignant mixed tumour (malignant chondroid syringoma).* Multinodular tumour including cystic structures

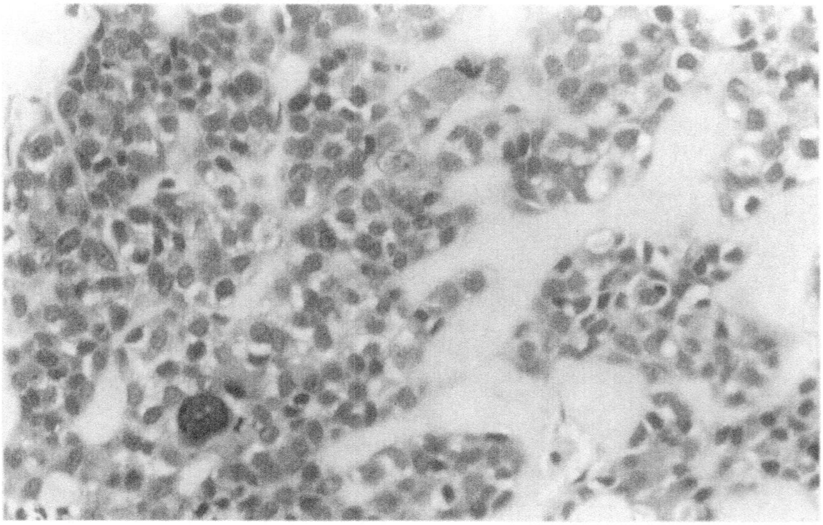

Fig. 69b. *Malignant mixed tumour (malignant chondroid syringoma).* Irregular groups of atypical cuboidal epithelium with pronounced nuclear pleomorphism embedded in chondroid stroma

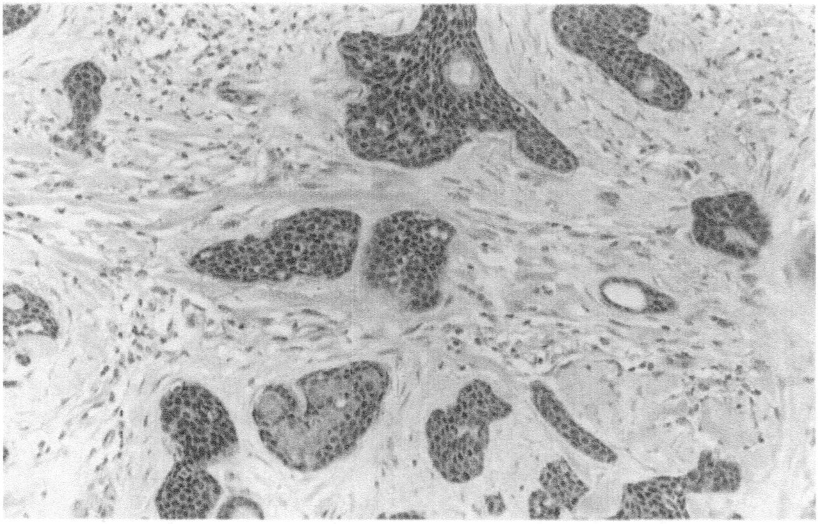

Fig. 70. *Porocarcinoma.* Infiltrating tumour composed of aggregates of atypical basaloid cells and larger atypical cells with pale cytoplasm. Several small ductal structures are present

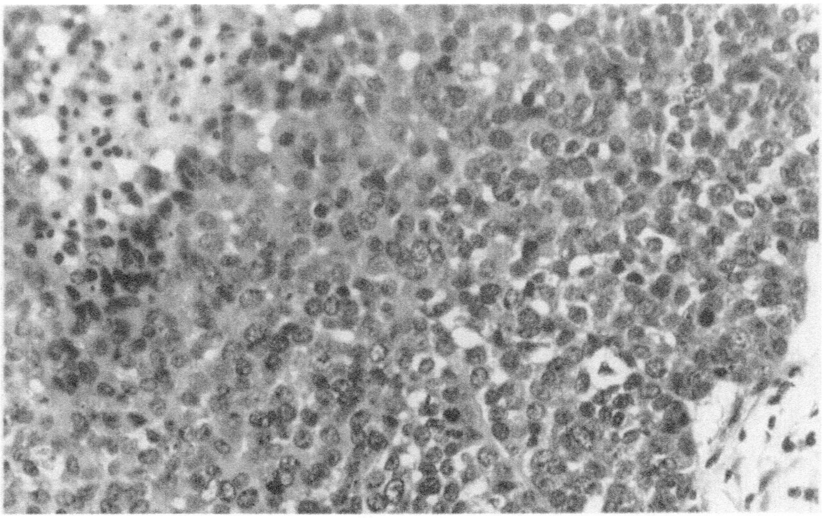

Fig. 71. *Malignant nodular hidradenoma.* Dense sheets of atypical polyhedral cells, scattered clear cells, mitoses and necrosis

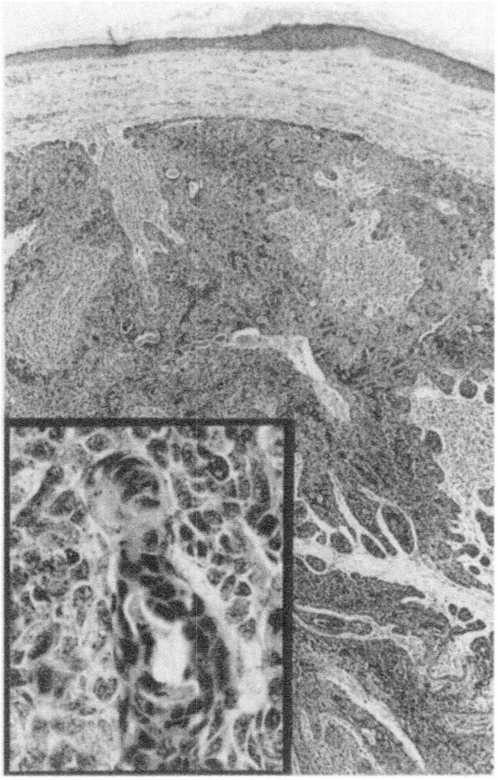

Fig. 72. *Malignant eccrine spiradenoma.* Nodules and sheets of atypical epithelial cells with foci of necrosis invade the deep dermis. *Inset*, small ductal structures are present

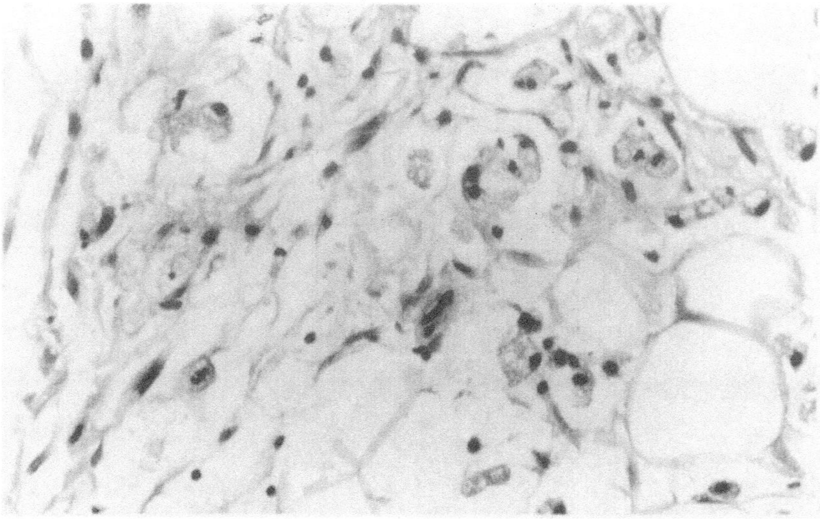

Fig. 73. *Mucinous eccrine carcinoma.* Solid clusters of large atypical epithelial cells with abundant cytoplasmic mucin and pleomorphic nuclei

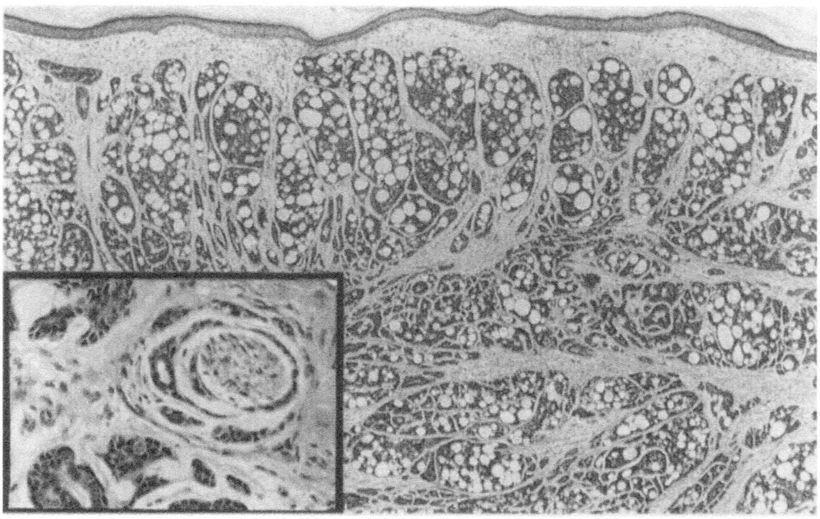

Fig. 74. *Adenoid cystic eccrine carcinoma.* Diffuse infiltration of the dermis by circumscribed solid and cystic groups of cells. *Inset*, small, solid and cystic groups of atypical basaloid cells embedded in fibrous stroma with a focus of perineural invasion

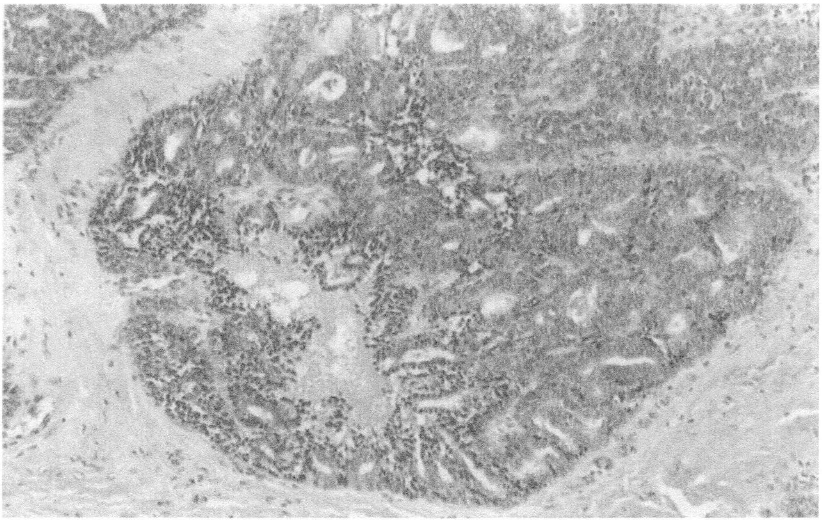

a

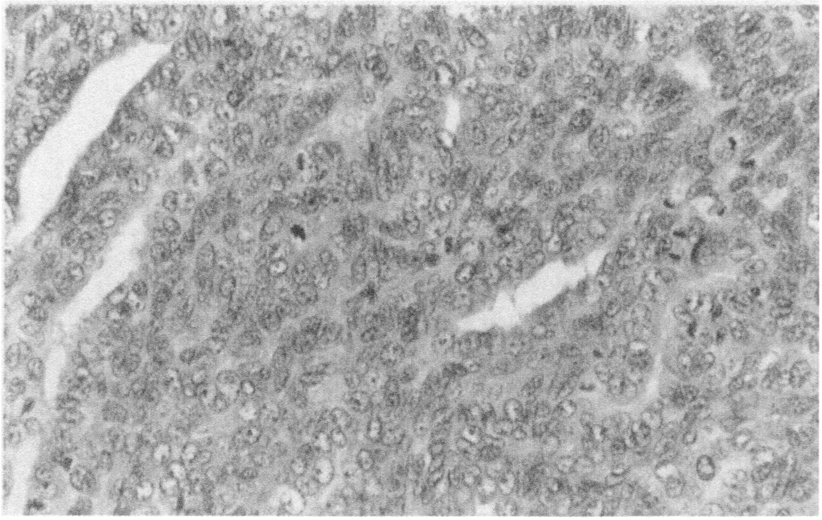

b

Fig. 75a,b. *Digital papillary adenocarcinoma.* **a** Central necrosis in a nodule including papillary and ductal structures. **b** Densely cellular zone of atypical cuboidal epithelium, with irregular ductal structures

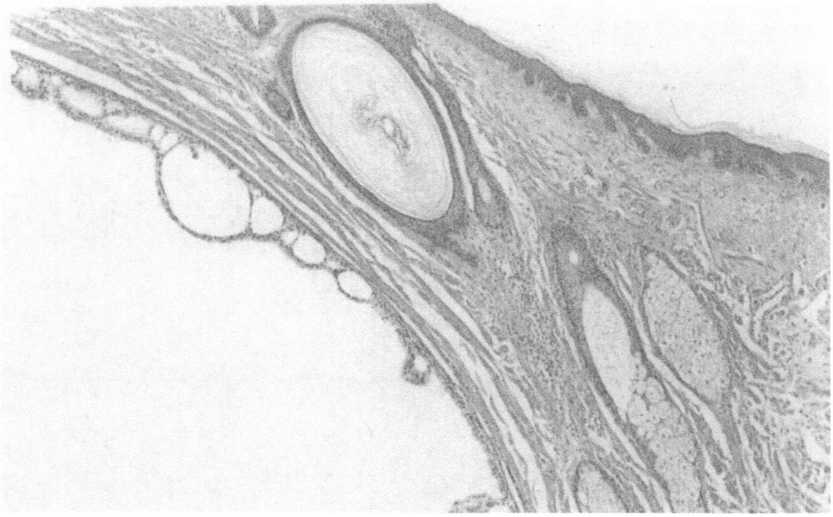

a

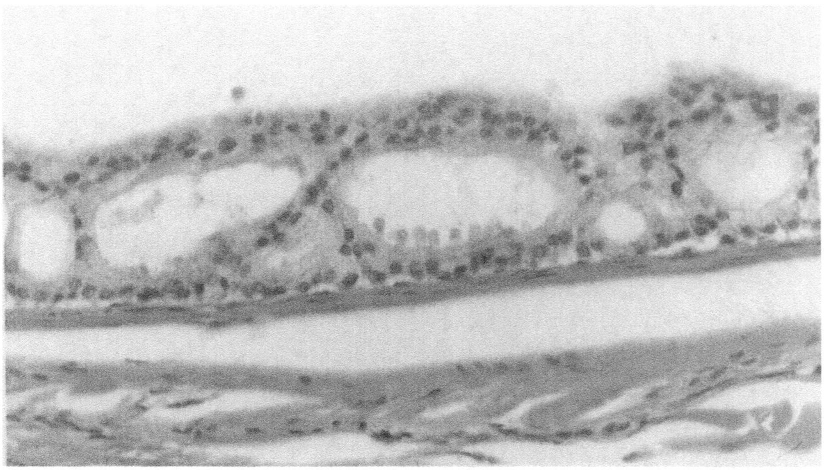

b

Fig. 76a,b. *Apocrine cystadenoma (hidrocystoma).* **a** A thin-walled cystic structure with small tufted epithelial projections. **b** Tufted projections lined by cuboidal and columnar epithelium with decapitation secretion

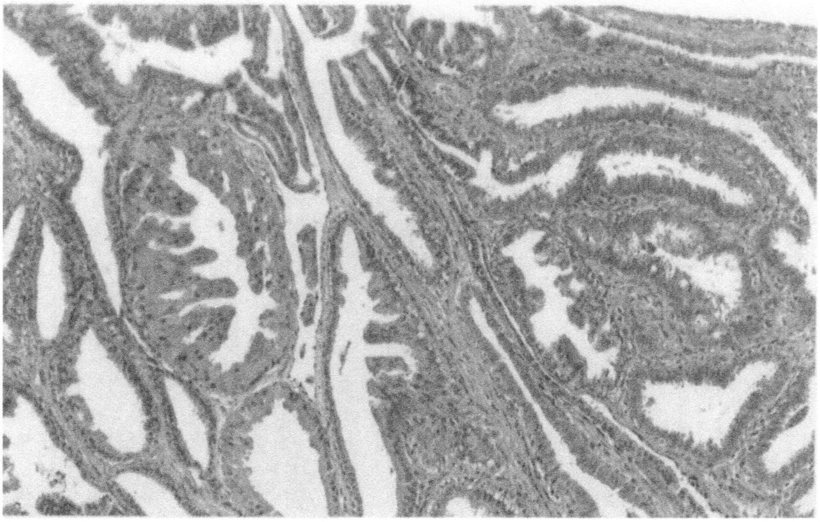

Fig. 77. *Hidradenoma papilliferum.* Cystic glandular spaces and papillary infoldings lined by columnar epithelium

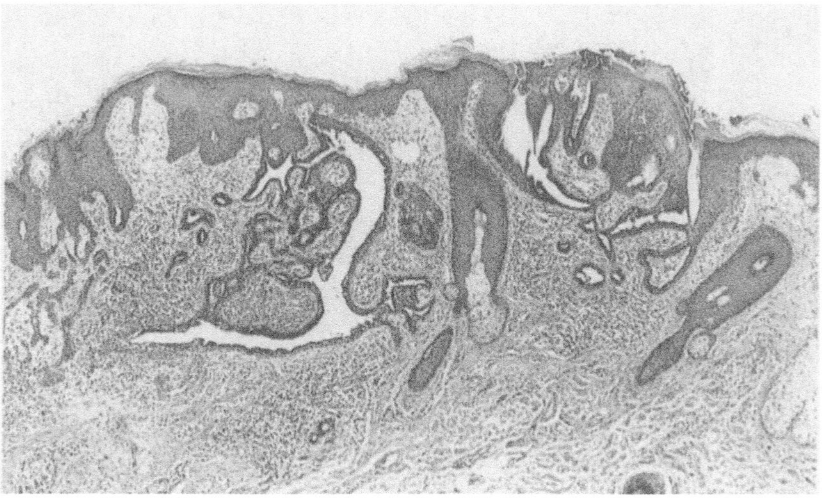

Fig. 78a. *Syringocystadenoma papilliferum.* Epidermal invaginations leading to ductal and cystic structures in the dermis

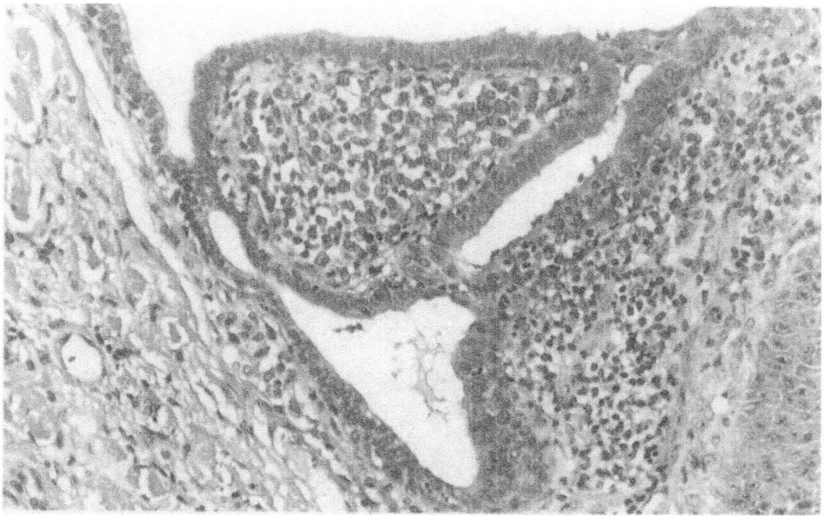

Fig. 78b. *Syringocystadenoma papilliferum.* Glandular structures are lined by columnar cells and basal cuboidal cells overlying stroma rich in plasma cells

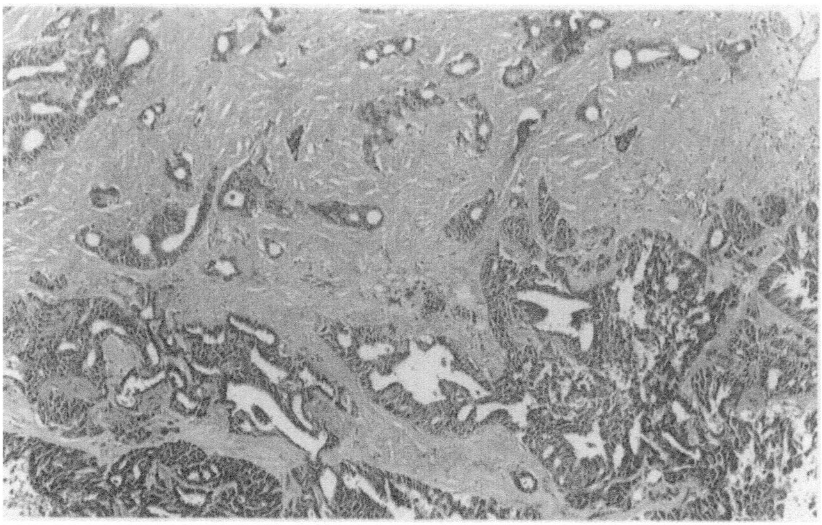

Fig. 79a. *Apocrine adenocarcinoma.* Infiltrating carcinoma composed of small ductal and larger cystic and cribriform structures

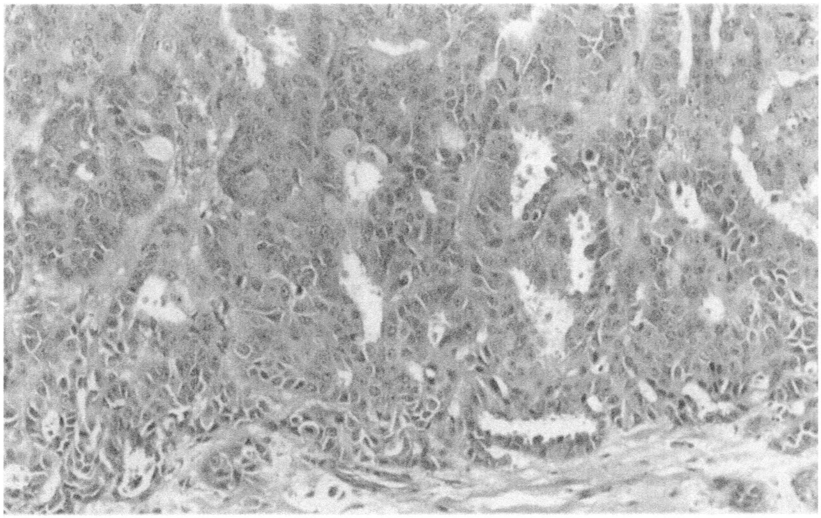

Fig. 79b. *Apocrine adenocarcinoma.* Densely packed atypical ductal structures lined by atypical columnar epithelium with focal decapitation secretion

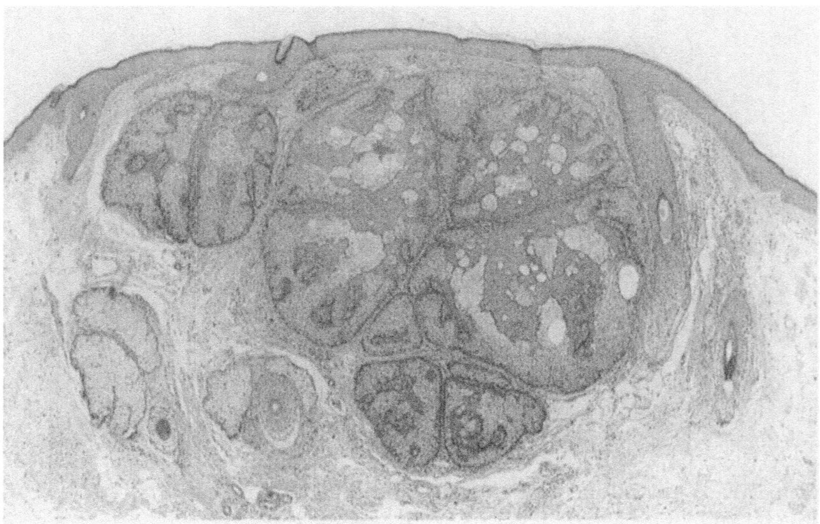

Fig. 80. *Sebaceous adenoma.* A circumscribed aggregate of large sebaceous glands

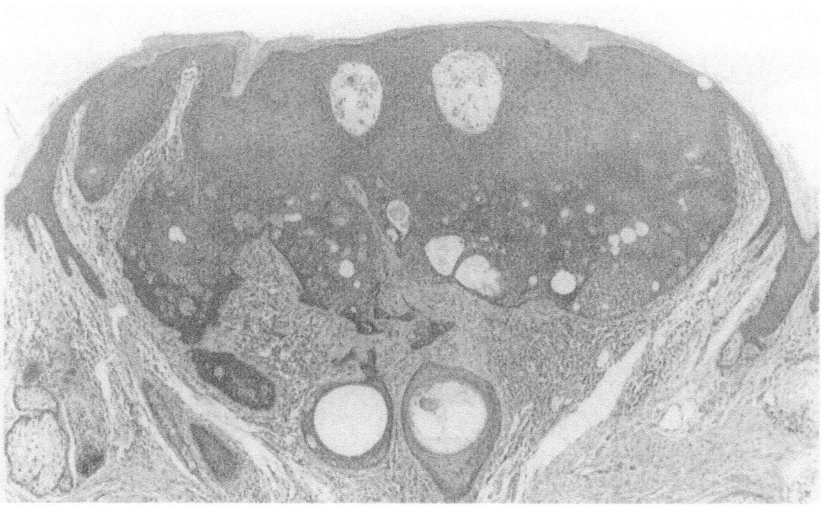

a

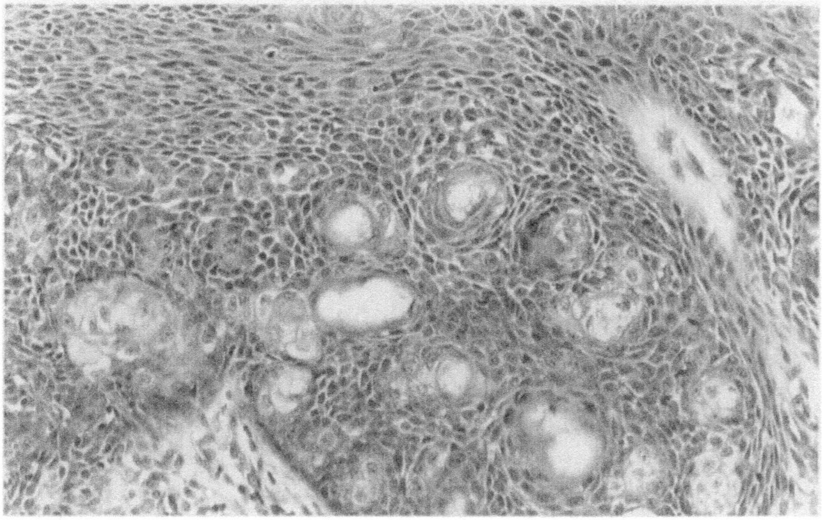

b

Fig. 81a,b. *Sebaceous epithelioma.* **a** Circumscribed lobules composed mainly of basaloid epithelium continuous with the epidermis. **b** Non-lipidized basaloid cells form the larger component of this lobule, in which there are small collections of lipidized sebaceous cells

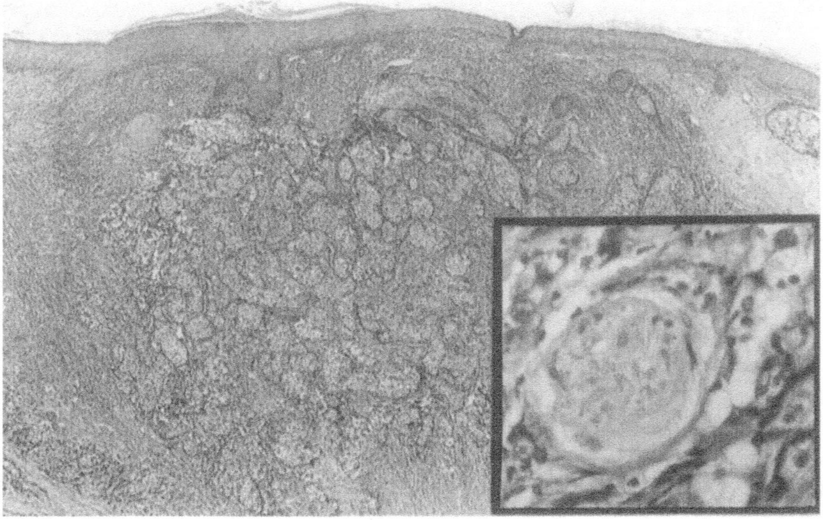

Fig. 82. *Sebaceous carcinoma.* Irregular lobules of sebaceous cells invading the dermis. *Inset*, atypical sebaceous cells with vacuolated cytoplasm, nuclear pleomorphism and perineural invasion

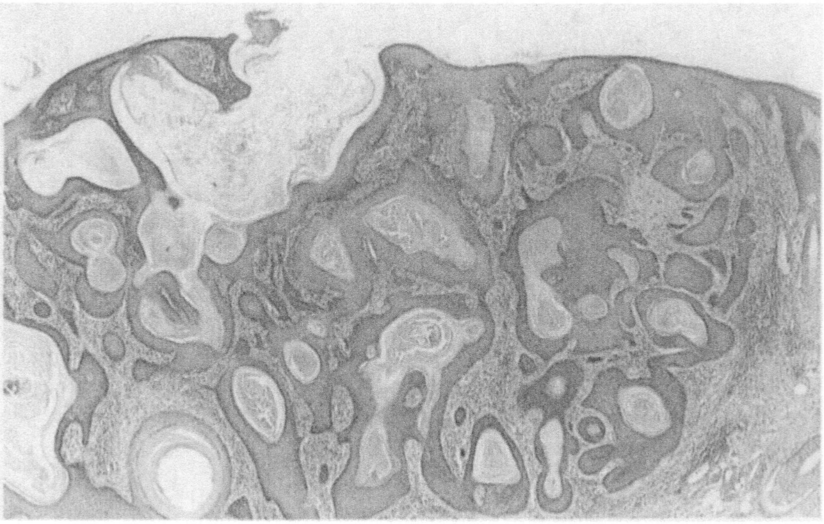

Fig. 83. *Naevus comedonicus.* Dilated follicular infundibula plugged with keratin

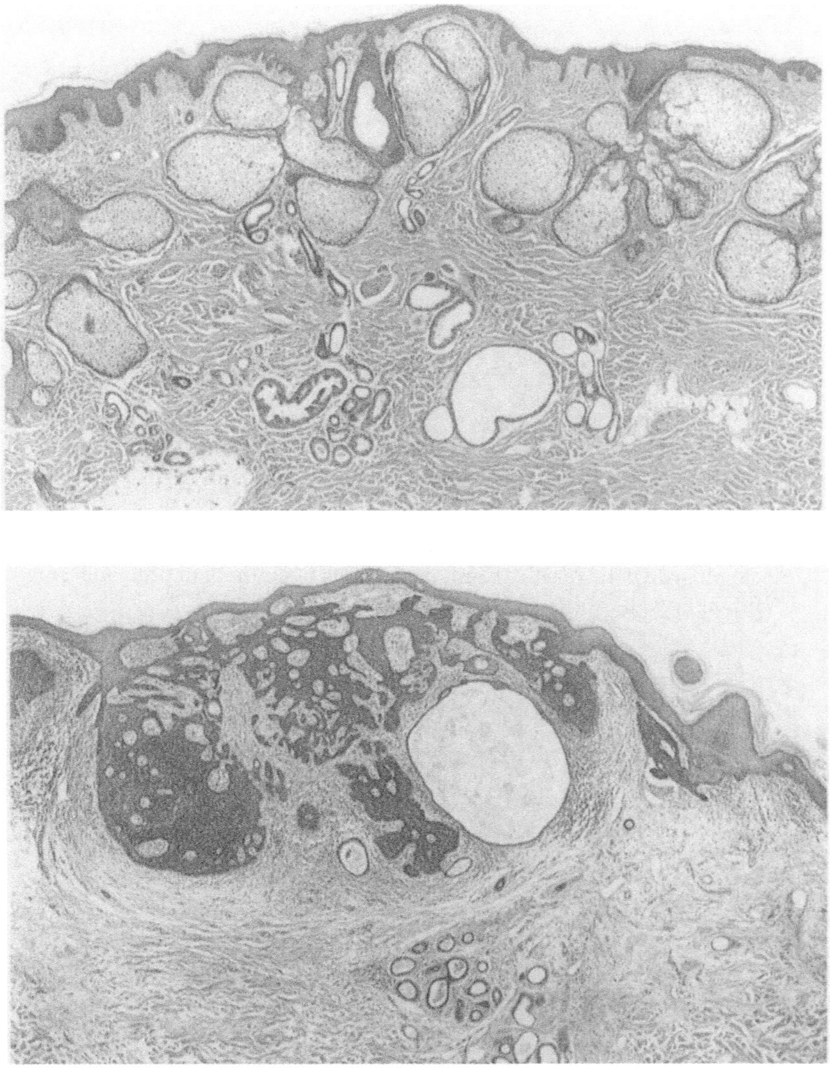

a

b

Fig. 84a,b. *Naevus sebaceus.* **a** Epidermal and sebaceous gland hyperplasia in association with ectopic apocrine glands. **b** Naevus sebaceus including basal cell carcinoma, apocrine glands and hidrocystoma-like cystic structures

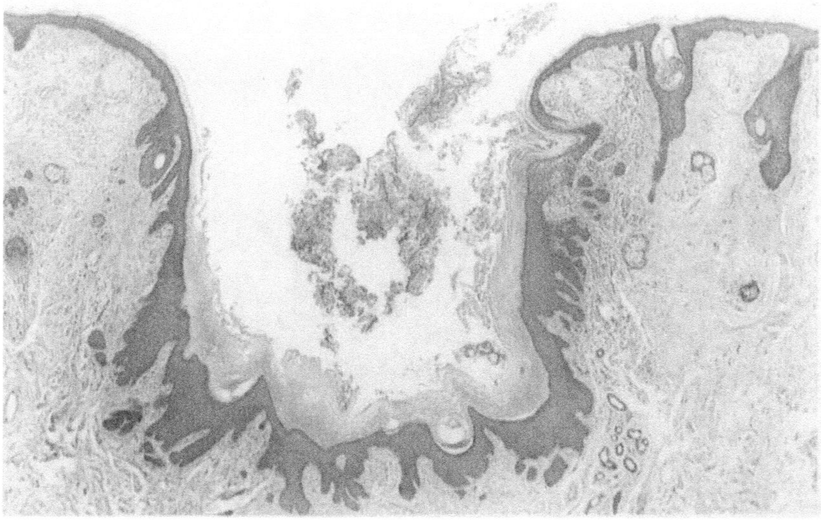

Fig. 85. *Conical infundibular acanthoma (dilated pore).* A widely dilated hair follicle plugged with keratin. Blunt projections of epithelium protrude from the infundibular wall

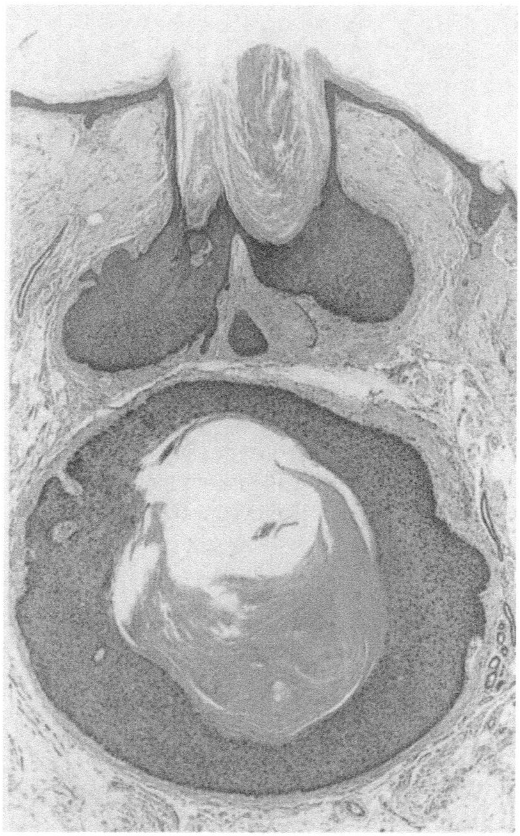

Fig. 86. *Pilar sheath acanthoma.* A dilated hair follicle ostium and infundibulum plugged with keratin overlie a cystic segment of hair follicle with a hyperplastic wall

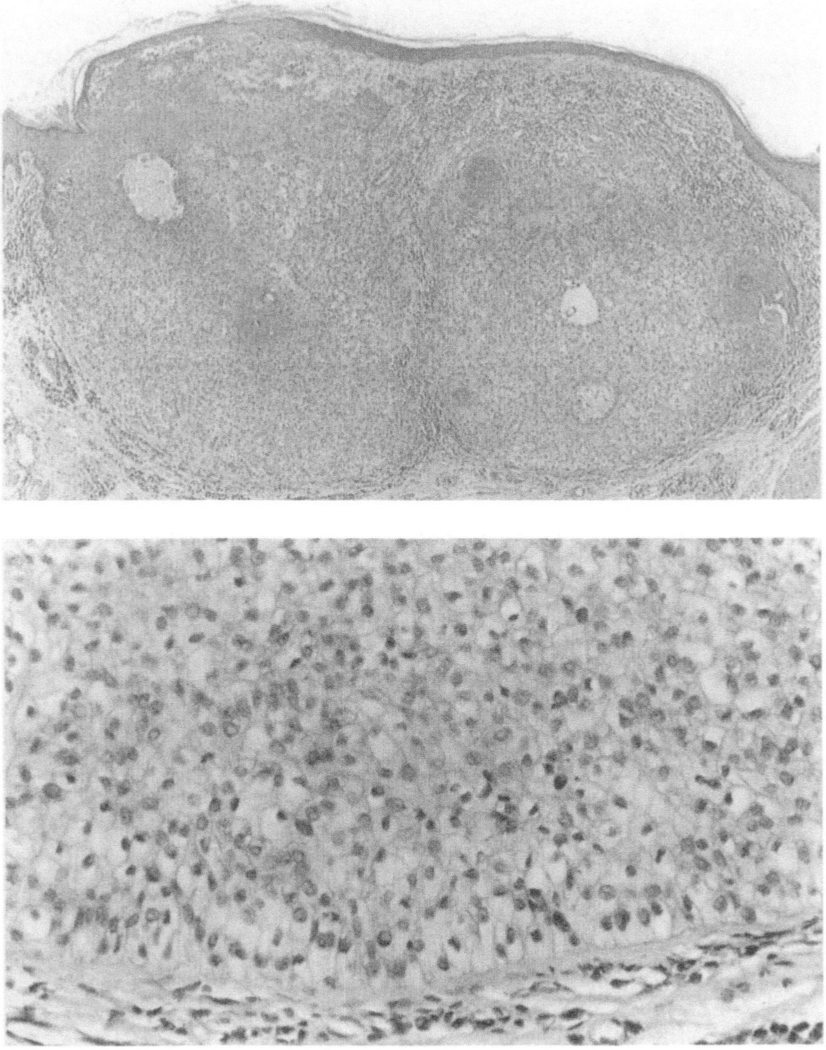

a

b

Fig. 87a,b. *Trichilemmoma.* **a** Circumscribed lobules continuous with the epidermis. **b** Peripheral palisades of columnar glycogenated epithelium overlying a prominent basement membrane

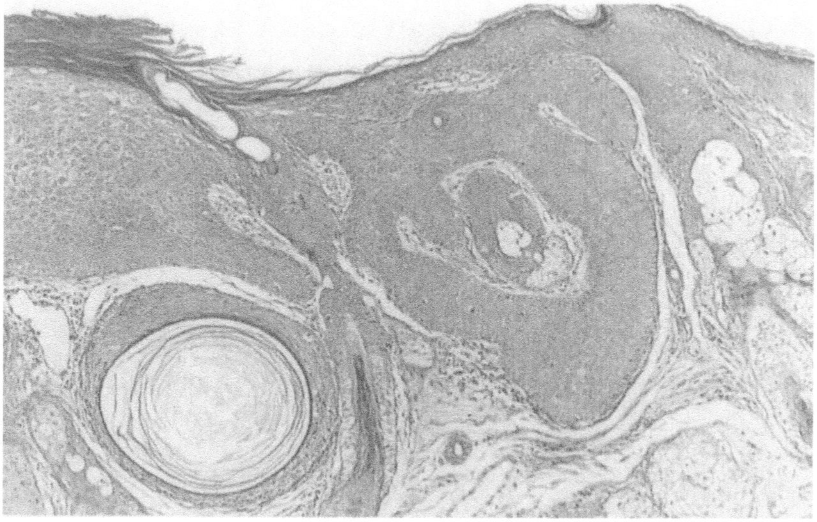

Fig. 88. *Tumour of follicular infundibulum.* Interlocking bands of squamous epithelium in the superficial dermis connected to the epidermis by slender bridges

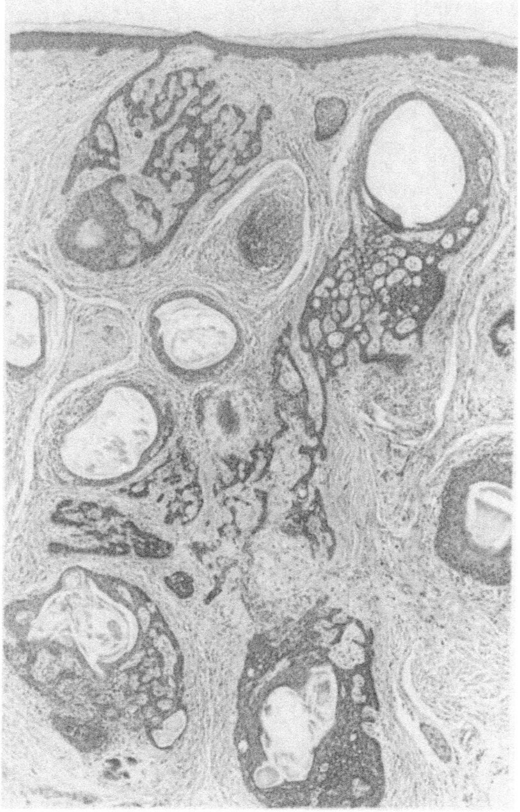

Fig. 89. *Trichoepithelioma.* Cribriform strands of basaloid cells and small keratinous cysts

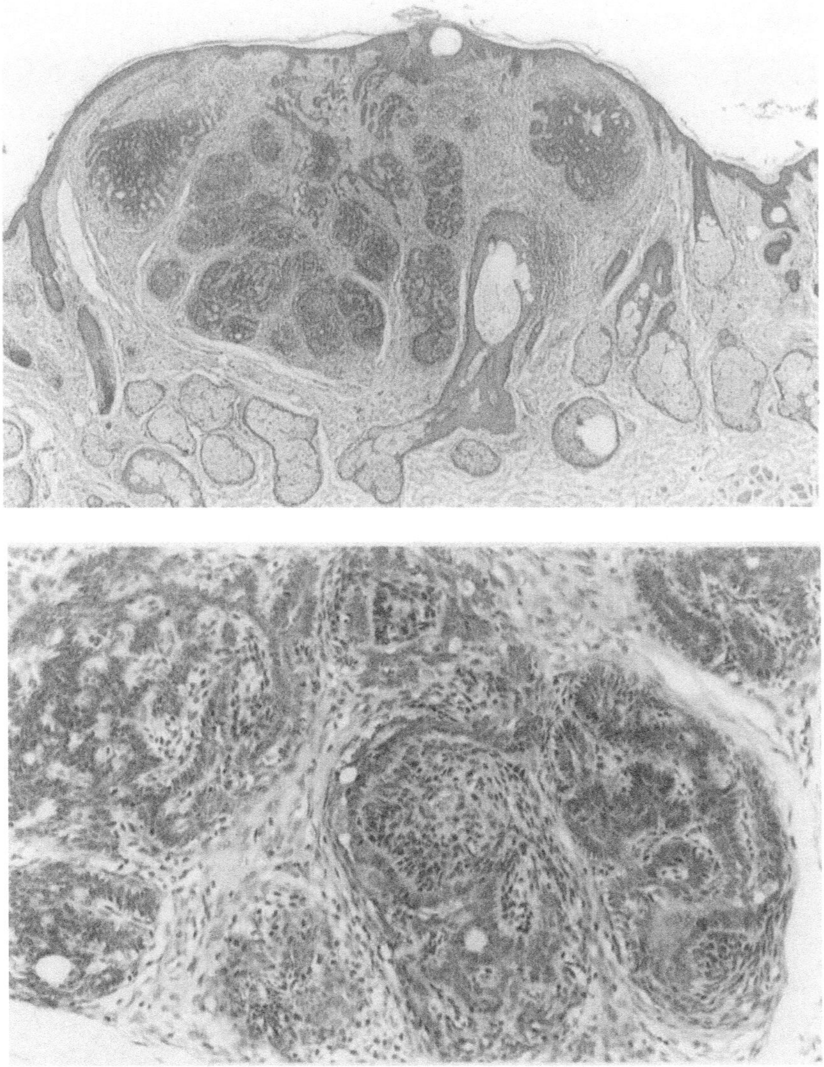

a

b

Fig. 90a,b. *Trichoblastoma.* **a** Lobulated tumour composed of cribriform strands of basaloid cells in a well-defined cellular stroma. **b** Lobules including primitive hair bulbs and papillae, and small cystic structures

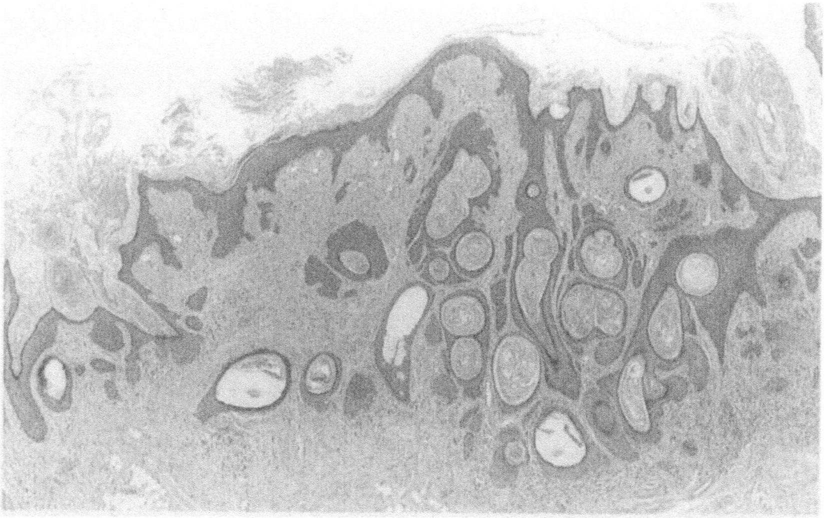

Fig. 91. *Trichoadenoma.* Predominant keratinous cysts with relatively little basaloid epithelioid component

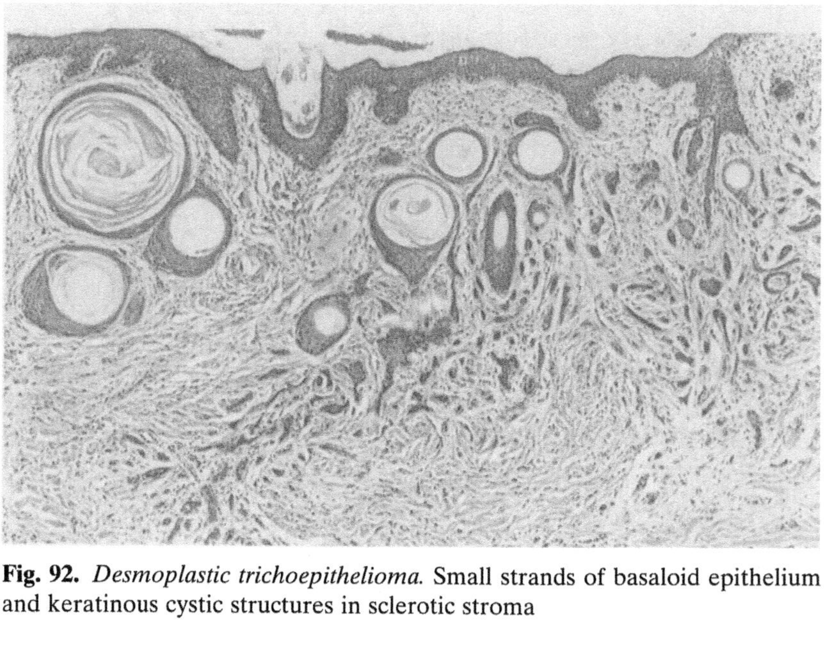

Fig. 92. *Desmoplastic trichoepithelioma.* Small strands of basaloid epithelium and keratinous cystic structures in sclerotic stroma

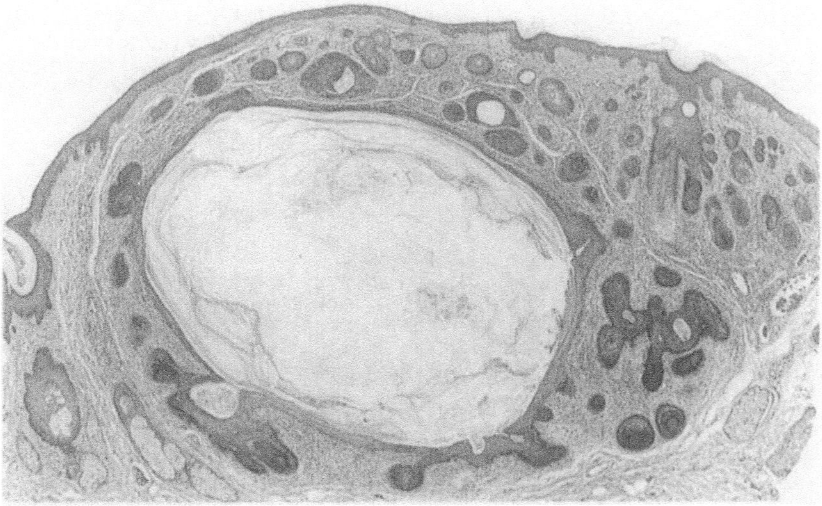

Fig. 93. *Trichofolliculoma.* A central cystically dilated hair follicle infundibulum from which small hair follicles project into the adjacent stroma

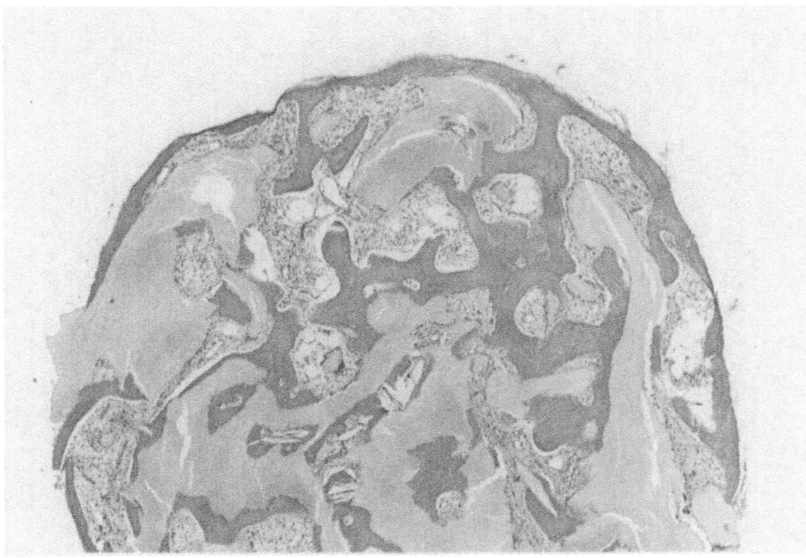

Fig. 94a. *Pilomatricoma.* Interlocking broad bands and sheets of basaloid epithelium merging with sheets of pale staining epithelium

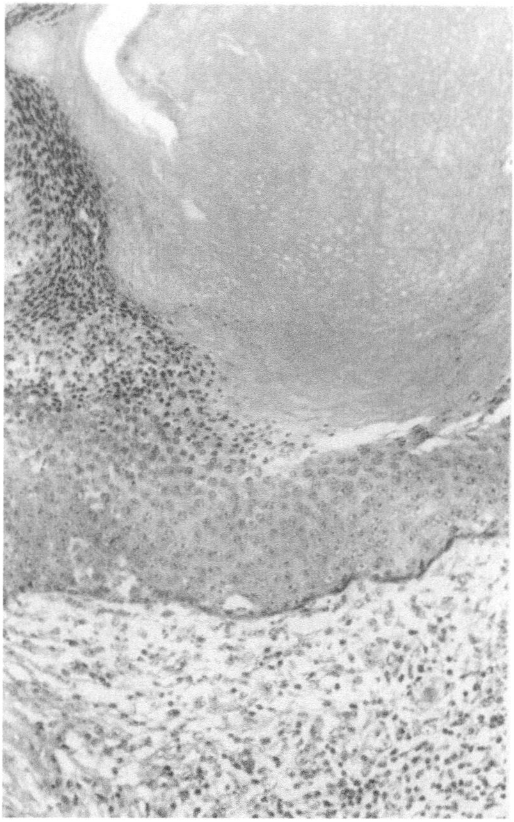

Fig. 94b. *Pilomatricoma.* Peripheral basaloid epithelium merging with shadow (ghost) cells

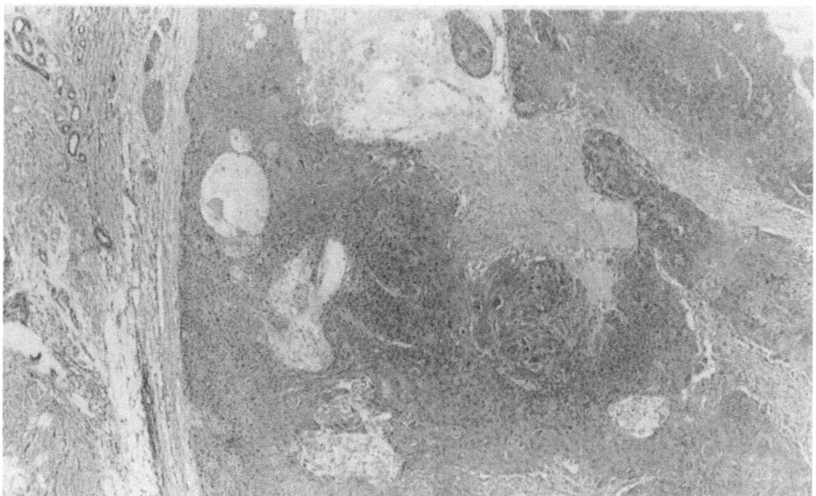

Fig. 95a. *Pilar tumour (proliferating trichilemmal cyst).* Sharply defined border and irregular ingrowths of squamoid epithelium pushing into the centre of the lesion, merging with dense keratin

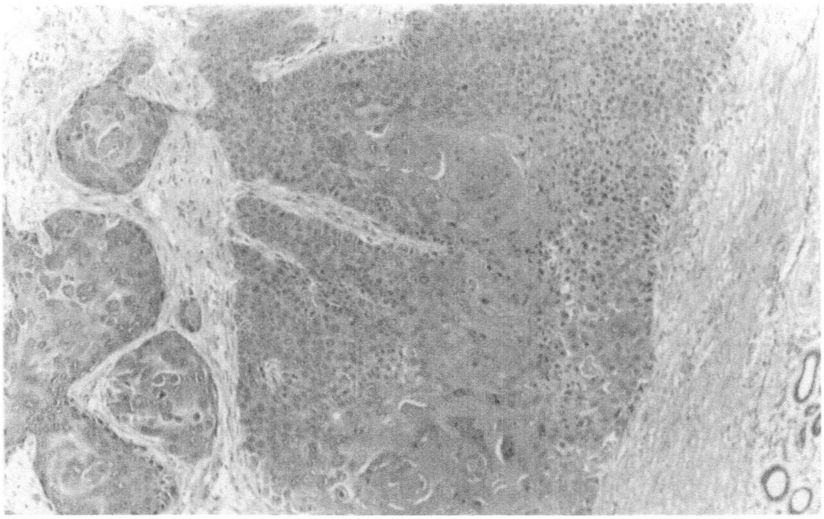

Fig. 95b. *Pilar tumour (proliferating trichilemmal cyst).* Broad bands and small nodules of large squamous and smaller basaloid cells with abrupt keratinization

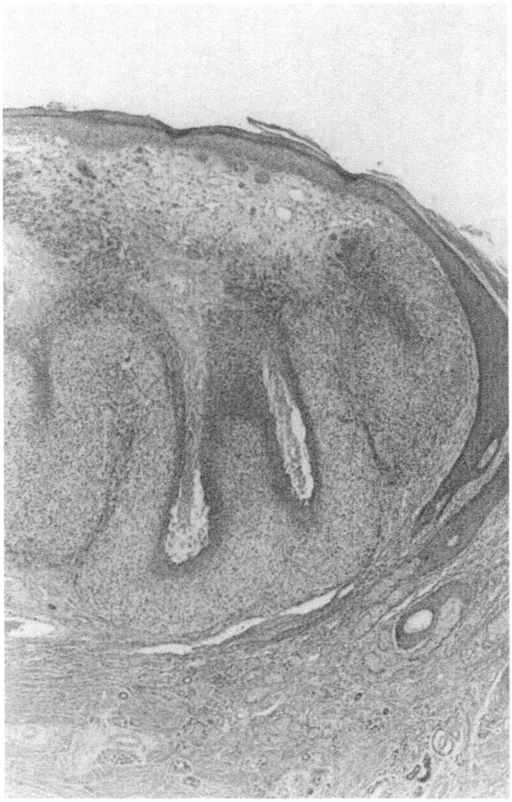

Fig. 96a. *Trichilemmo-carcinoma.* Circumscribed tumour composed of interconnecting lobules of clear and pale cells

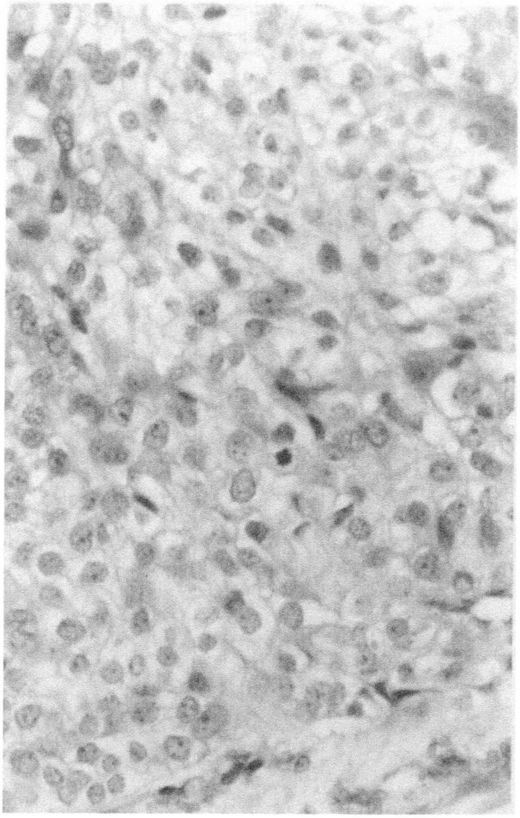

Fig. 96b. *Trichilemmo-carcinoma.* Atypical clear cells with pleomorphic nuclei and occasional mitoses

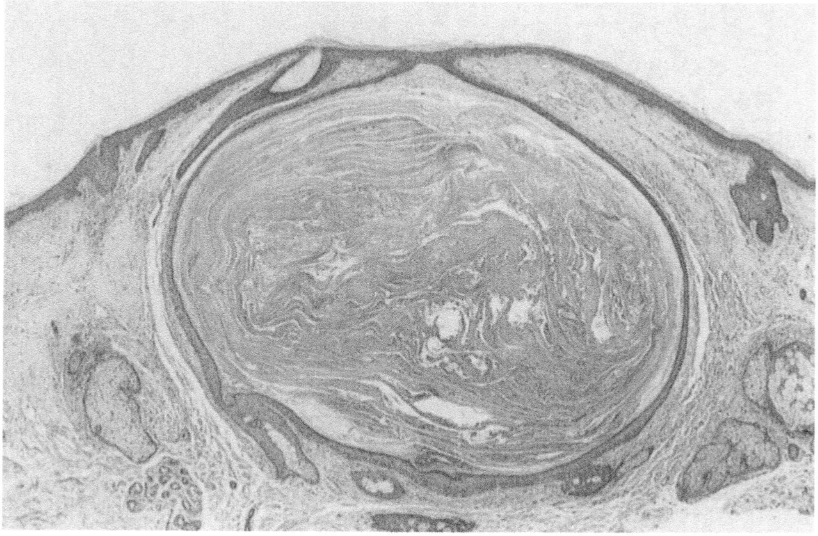

Fig. 97. *Infundibular cyst.* A thin walled cyst lined by stratified squamous epithelium, containing laminated keratin. Two small hair follicles are attached to the base of the cyst

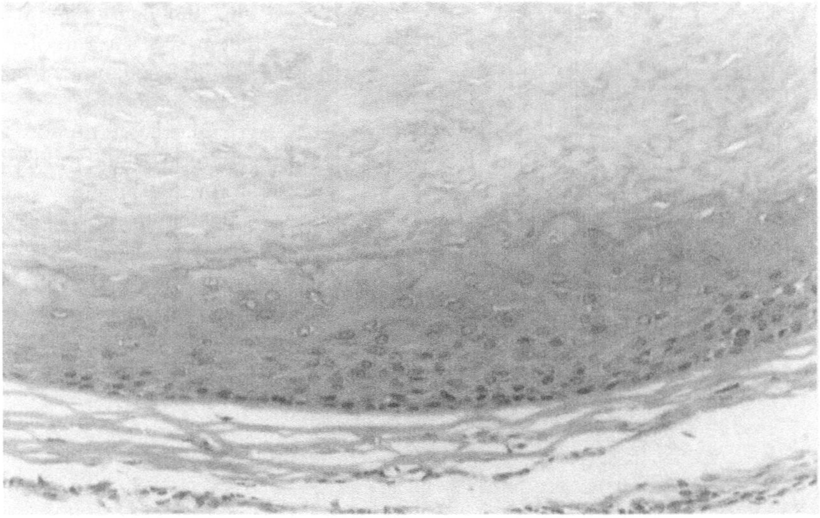

Fig. 98. *Trichilemmal cyst (pilar cyst).* The wall of squamous epithelium has no granular layer

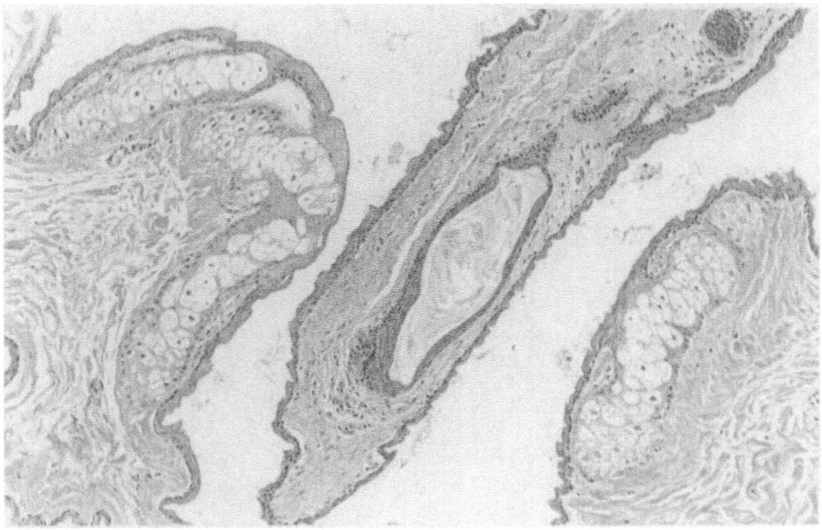

Fig. 99. *Steatocystoma multiplex.* Undulating wall of squamous epithelium with attached lobules of sebaceous glands

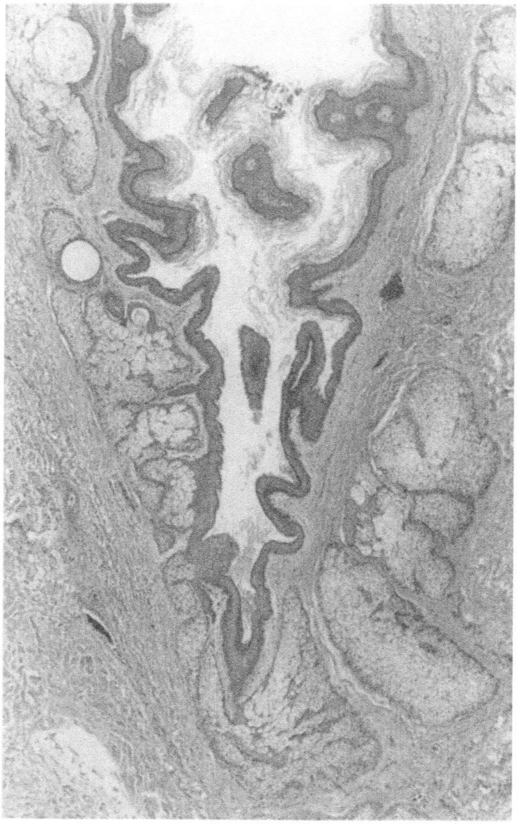

Fig. 100. *Dermoid cyst.* The cyst has a wall of stratified squamous epithelium with a granular layer; numerous sebaceous gland lobules are present in the adjacent stroma

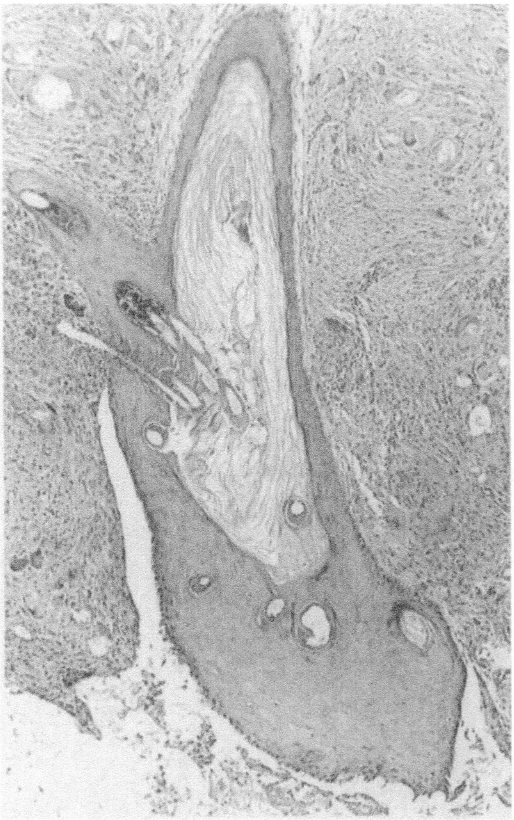

Fig. 101. *Eruptive vellus hair cyst.* The cyst contains keratin and numerous small segments of hair shaft

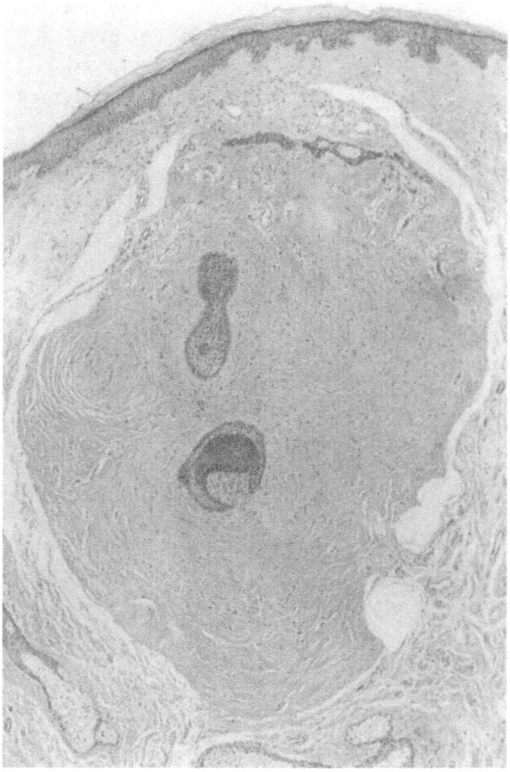

Fig. 102. *Perifollicular fibroma.* Compact cellular fibrous tissue surrounds segments of hair follicle

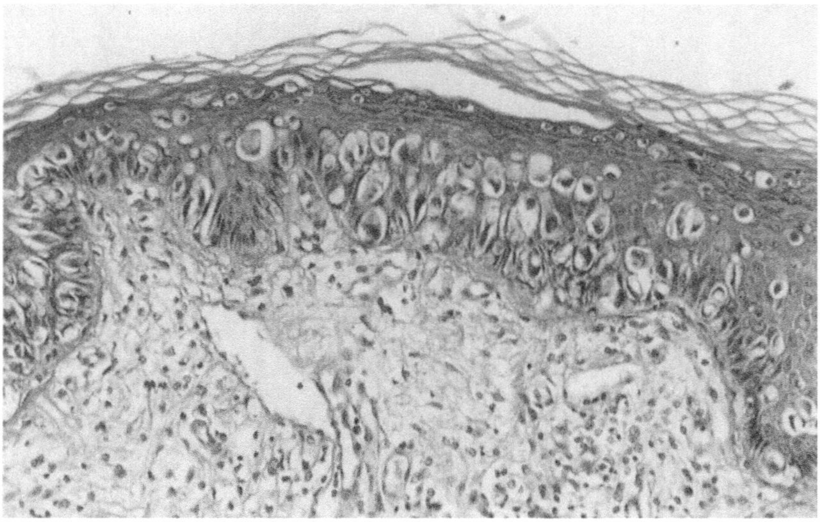

Fig. 103. *Extramammary Paget disease.* Atypical epithelial cells with pale or clear cytoplasm infiltrate the full thickness of the epidermis

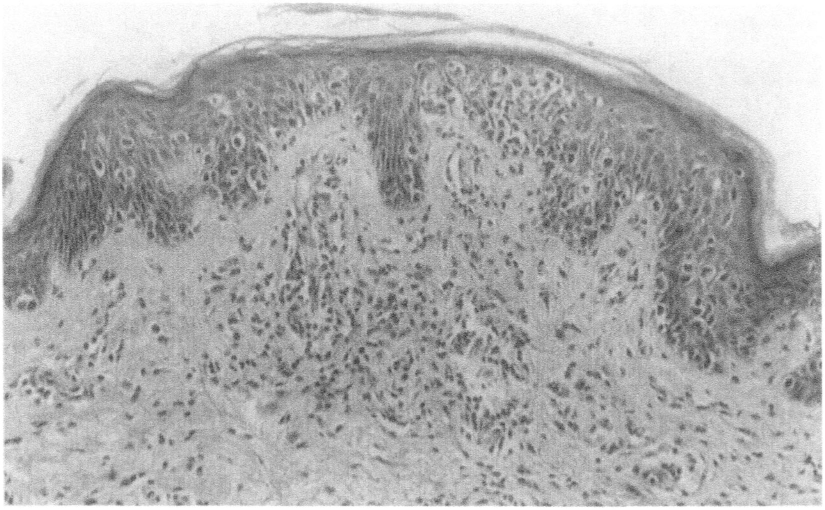

a

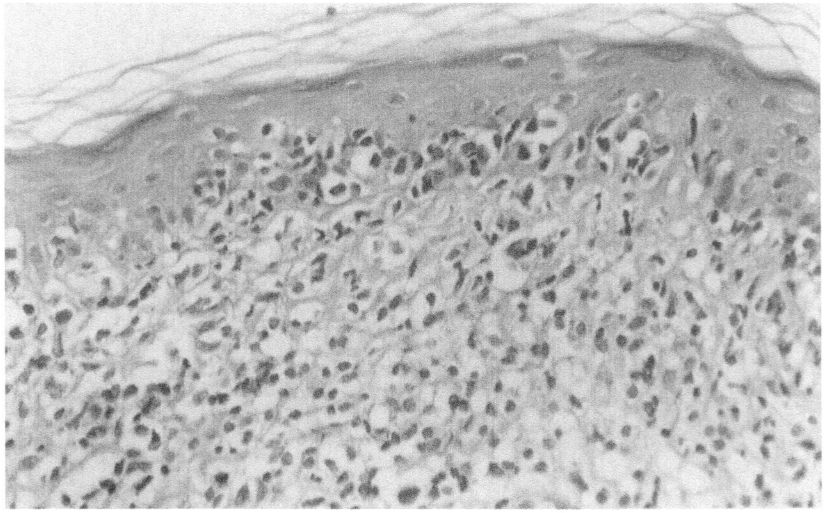

b

Fig. 104a,b. *Mycosis fungoides.* **a** Extensive epidermotropism of the hyperplastic epidermis by pleomorphic lymphocytes associated with little or no spongiosis. **b** Pleomorphic lymphocytes arranged singly and in small groups (Pautrier microabscesses) in lacunar spaces in the epidermis

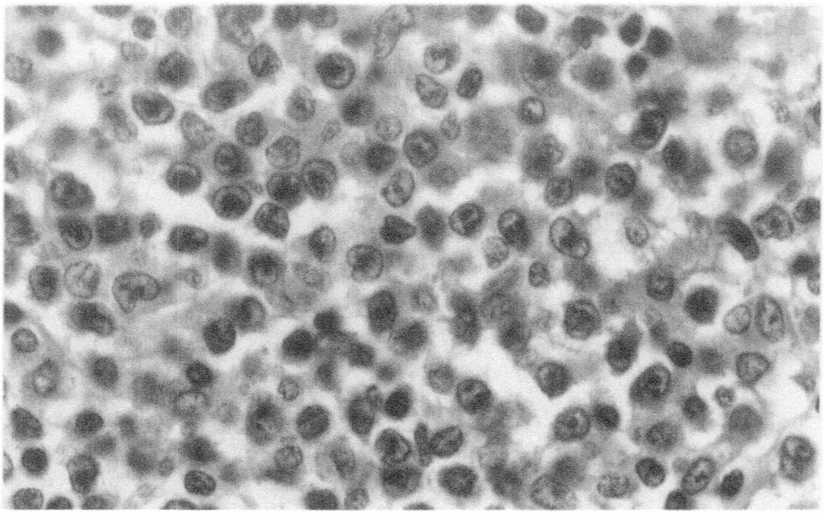

c

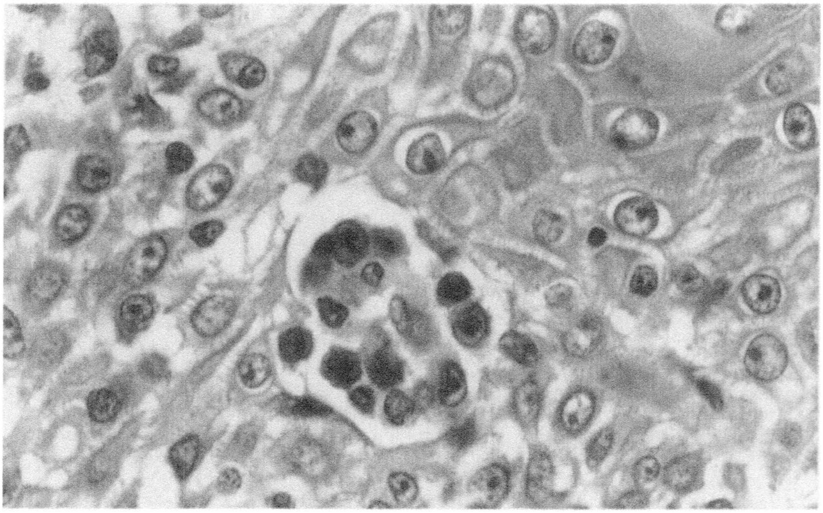

d

Fig. 104c,d. *Mycosis fungoides.* **c** Indented and convoluted nuclear membranes of atypical T lymphocytes in mycosis fungoides (B5 fixation). **d** Intra-epidermal collection of atypical lymphocytes (Pautrier microabscesses)

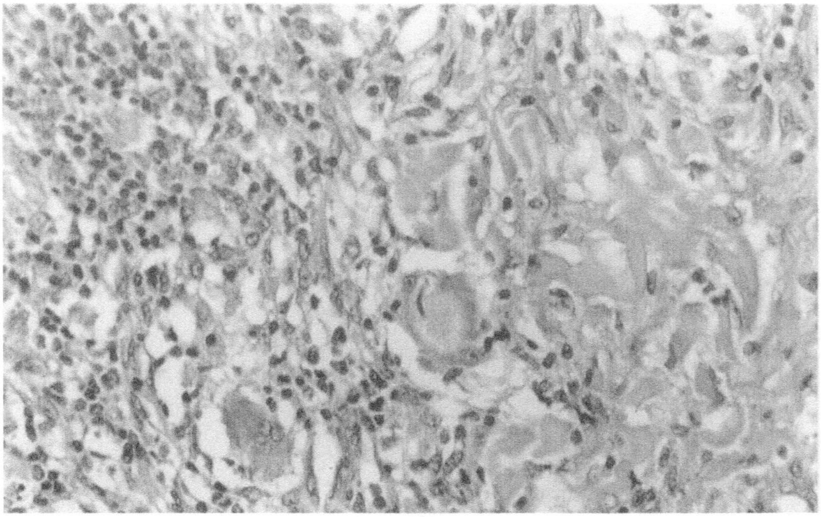

Fig. 105. *Granulomatous slack skin.* Elastophagocytosis by macrophages and giant cells associated with a diffuse atypical lymphocytic infiltrate

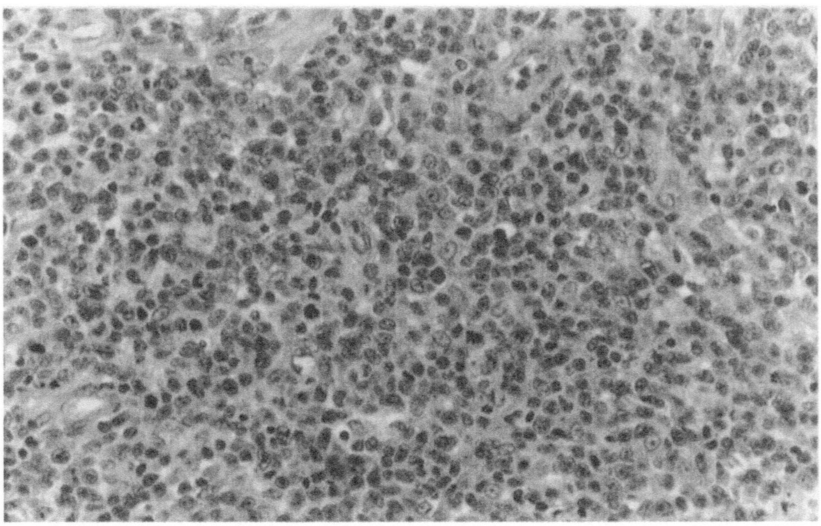

Fig. 106. *Cutaneous B cell lymphoma.* Diffuse dermal infiltration by small lymphocytes and large, atypical lymphocytes with hyperchromatic nuclei

a
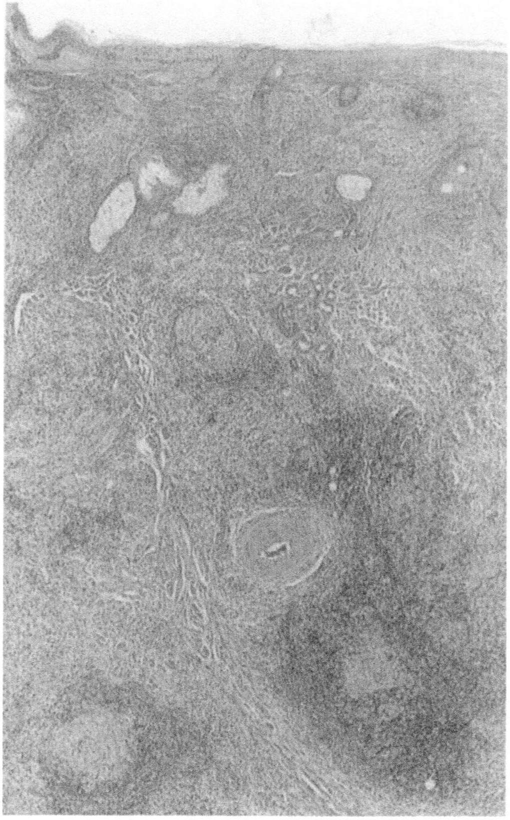

b
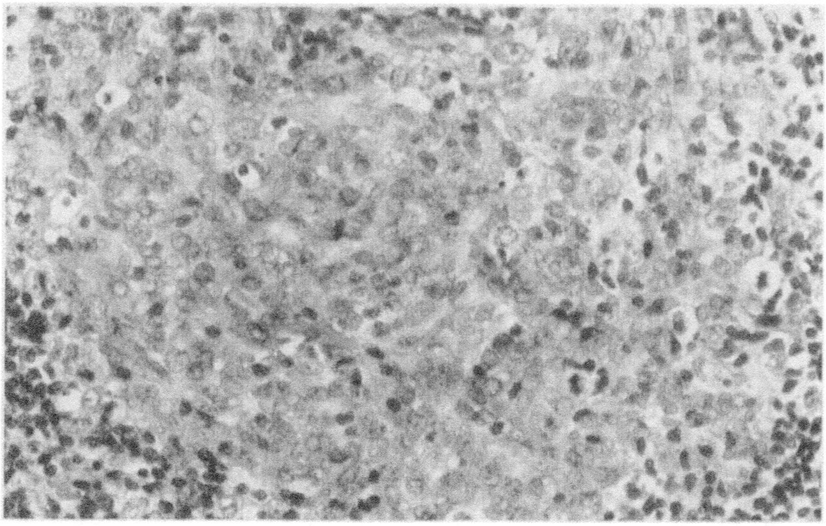

Fig. 107a,b. *Primary cutaneous follicular lymphoma.* **a** Deep and dense dermal lymphocytic infiltrate including irregular follicular structures in the deeper layers. **b** Monomorphic population within a follicle, no tingible body macrophages and only a thin follicular mantle

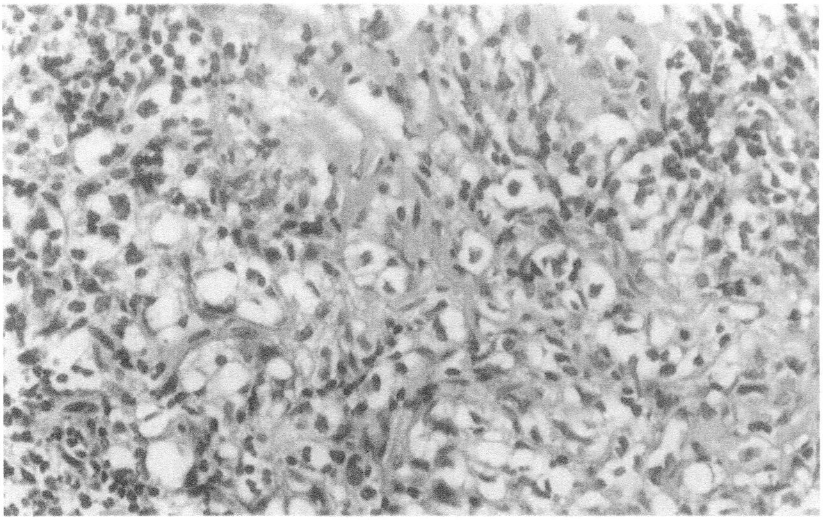

Fig. 107c. *Primary cutaneous follicular lymphoma.* Atypical lymphocytes with ballooned, clear cytoplasm

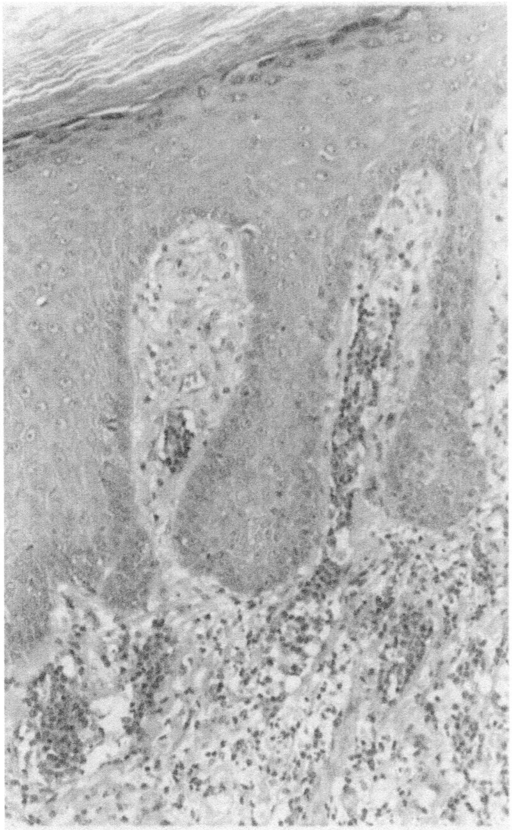

Fig. 108. *Malignant angioendotheliomatosis.* Atypical lymphoid cells in dilated dermal blood vessels

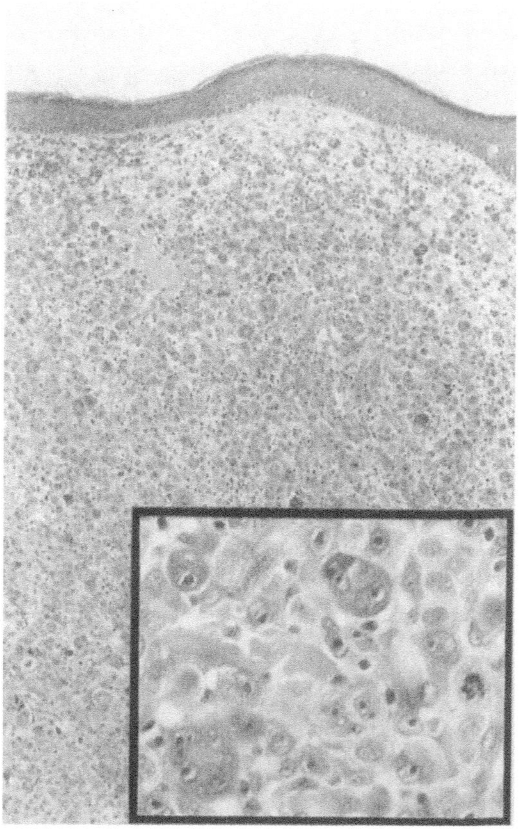

Fig. 109. *Large cell anaplastic lymphoma.* Deep and diffuse dermal infiltration by large atypical cells with pale cytoplasm. The epidermis is not infiltrated. *Inset,* the neoplastic cells have abundant pale cytoplasm and large ovoid or round nuclei with prominent nucleoli. Mitoses and giant cells are present

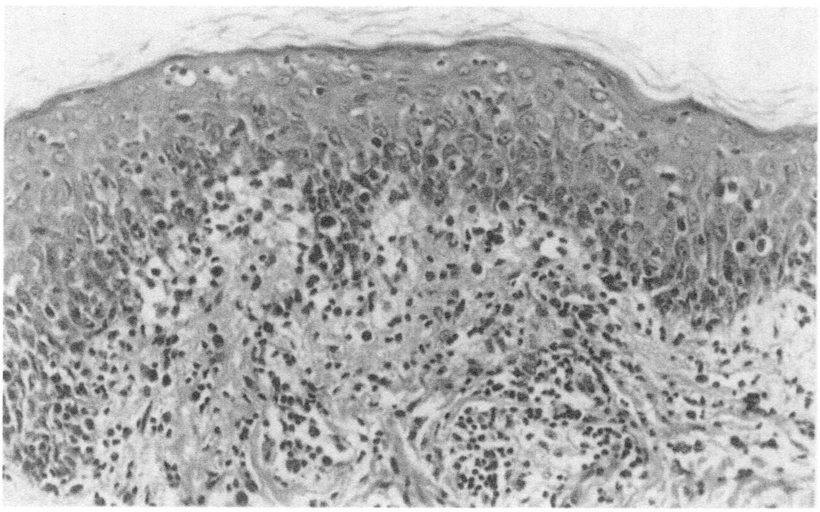

Fig. 110. *Lymphomatoid papulosis.* Superficial dermal infiltration by pleomorphic atypical lymphoid cells; epidermal infiltration by atypical lymphocytes arranged singly

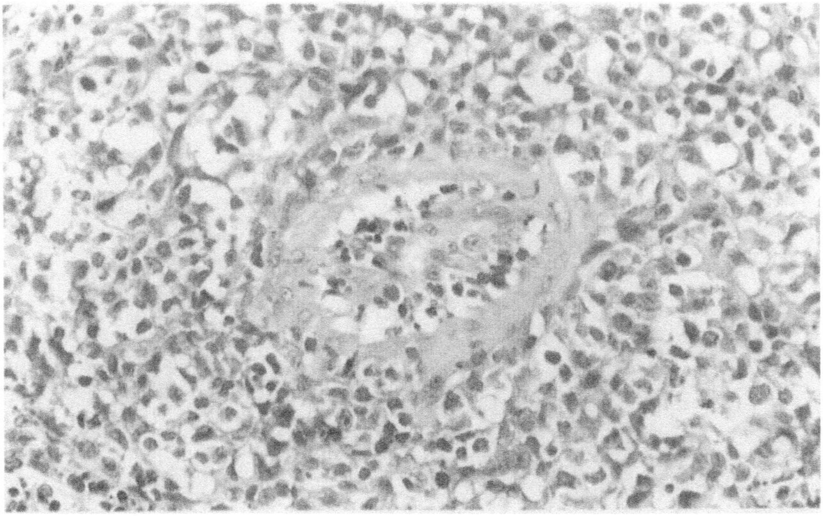

Fig. 111. *Lymphomatoid granulomatosis.* Infiltration of blood vessel wall by atypical lymphocytes

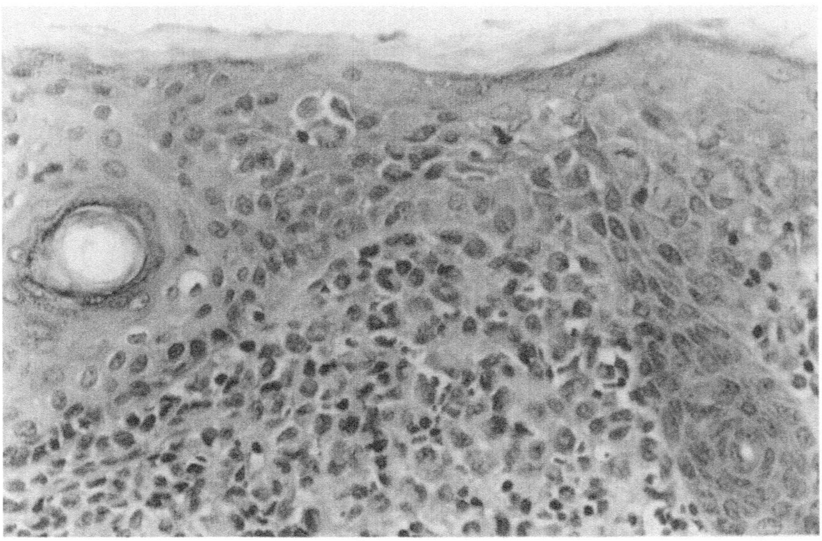

Fig. 112. *Langerhans cell histiocytosis (histiocytosis X).* Dermal invasion and focal epidermal infiltration by atypical mononuclear cells with abundant pale cytoplasm and indented nuclei

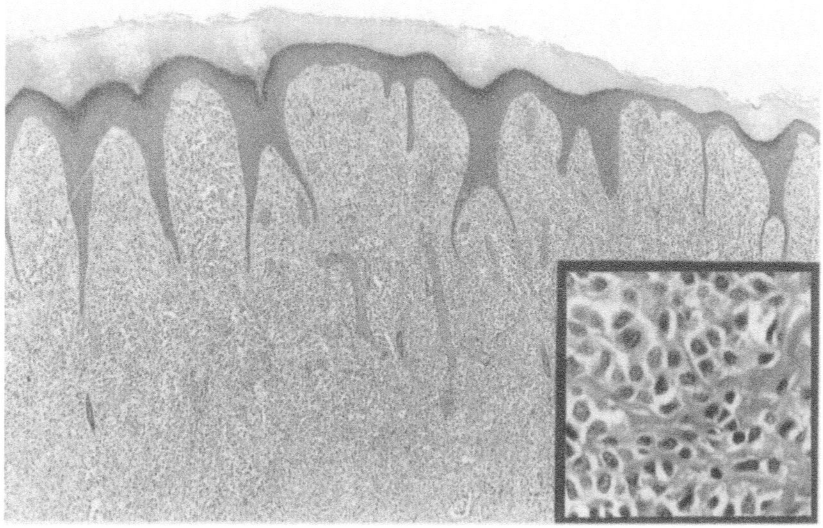

Fig. 113. *Mastocytoma.* Hyperplastic epidermis overlies a dense, diffuse dermal mononuclear cellular infiltrate. *Inset*, the infiltrating cells have granular cytoplasm and central ovoid or round nuclei

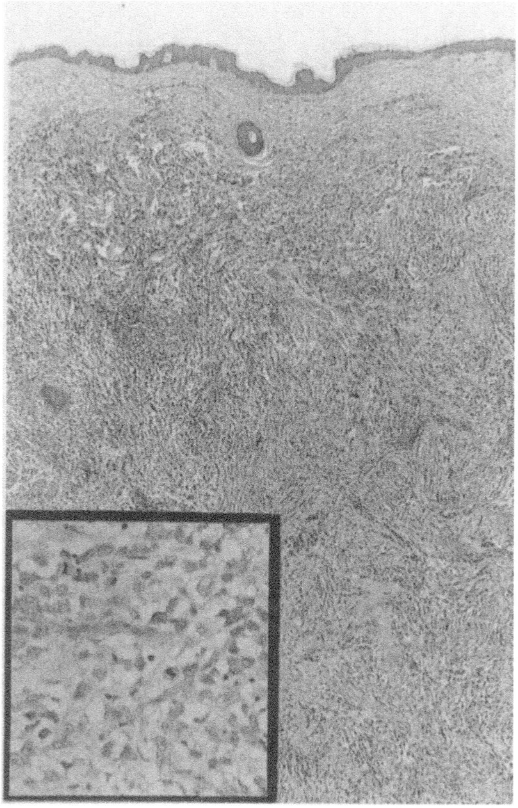

Fig. 114. *Leukaemia cutis.* A grenz zone separates the epidermis from a diffuse dermal infiltrate of mononuclear cells. *Inset*, atypical myeloid cells with numerous mitoses

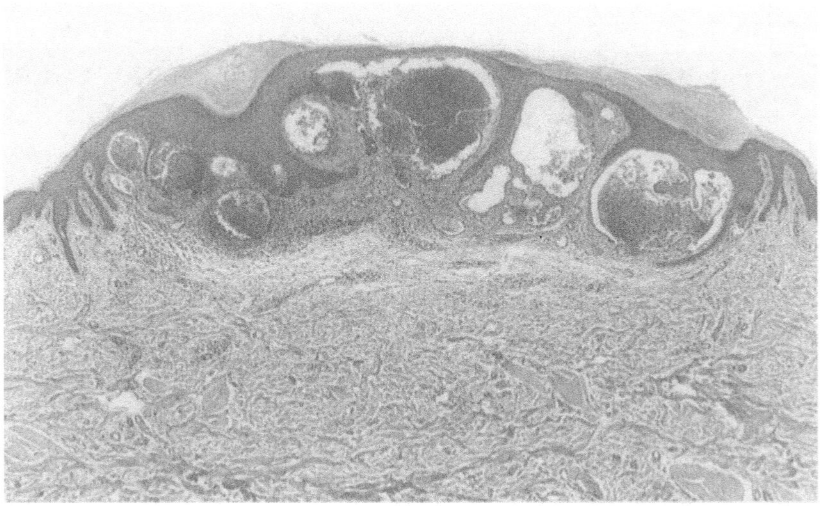

Fig. 115. *Angiokeratoma.* Elongated rete ridges form collarettes around dilated blood vessels in the papillary dermis

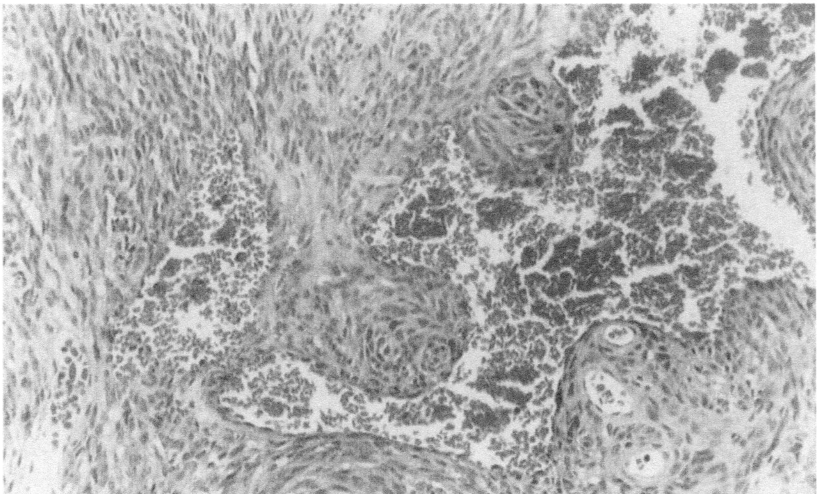

Fig. 116. *Tufted haemangioma.* Invaginations of plump spindle-shaped, pericyte-like cells bulge into the lumina of blood vessels

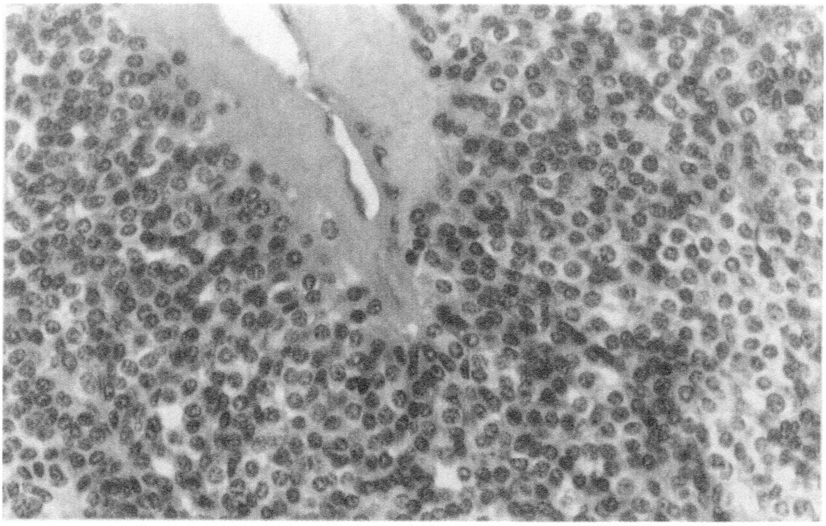

Fig. 117. *Glomus tumour.* Densely packed uniform cells with central round nuclei surround a blood vessel

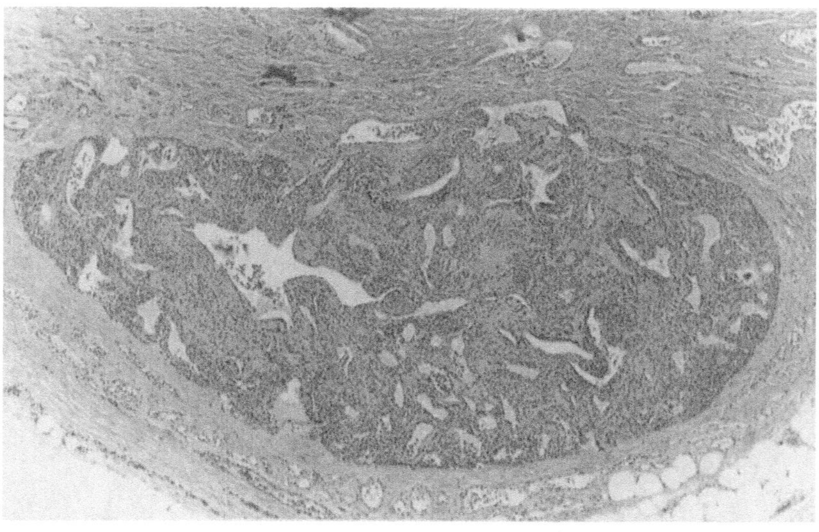

Fig. 118. *Glomangioma.* Circumscribed nodular tumour with compact small cells surrounding blood vessels of irregular size and shape

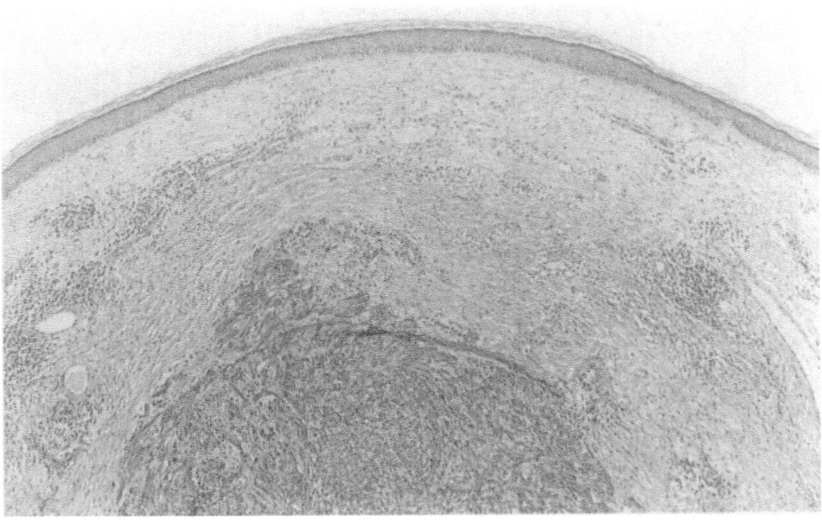

a

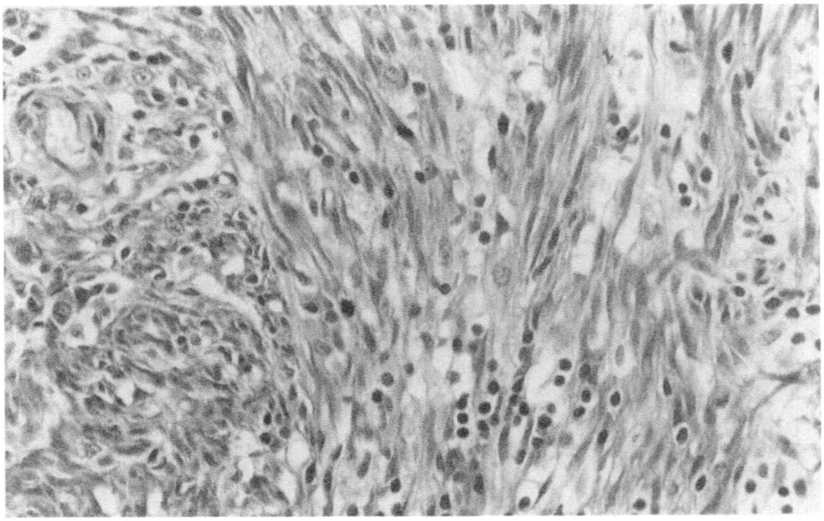

b

Fig. 119a,b. *Kaposi sarcoma.* **a** Nodular stage, showing dermal infiltration by irregular nodules. **b** Fascicles of spindle cells with hyperchromatic nuclei, slit-like spaces containing erythrocytes and scattered lymphocytes between the spindle cells

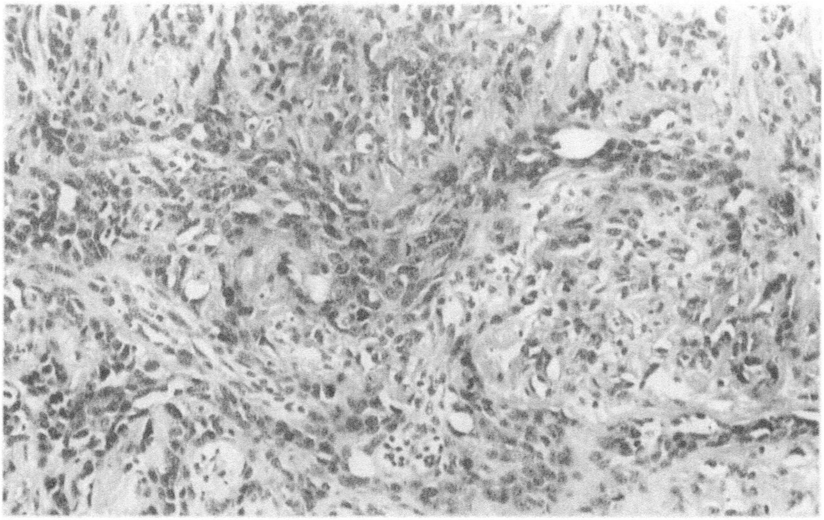

Fig. 120. *Angiosarcoma.* Aggregates of atypical endothelial cells and spindle cells surround irregular vascular spaces

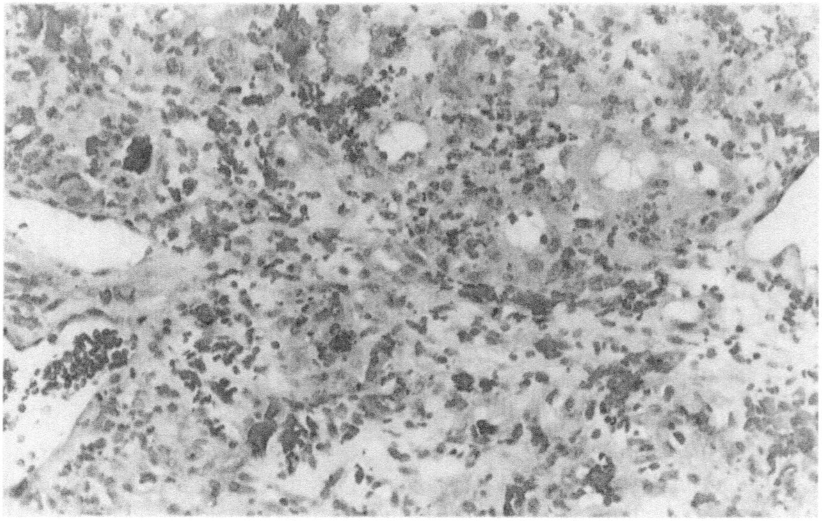

Fig. 121. *Bacillary angiomatosis.* Lobular collections of small blood vessels with plump endothelial cells embedded in an oedematous stroma

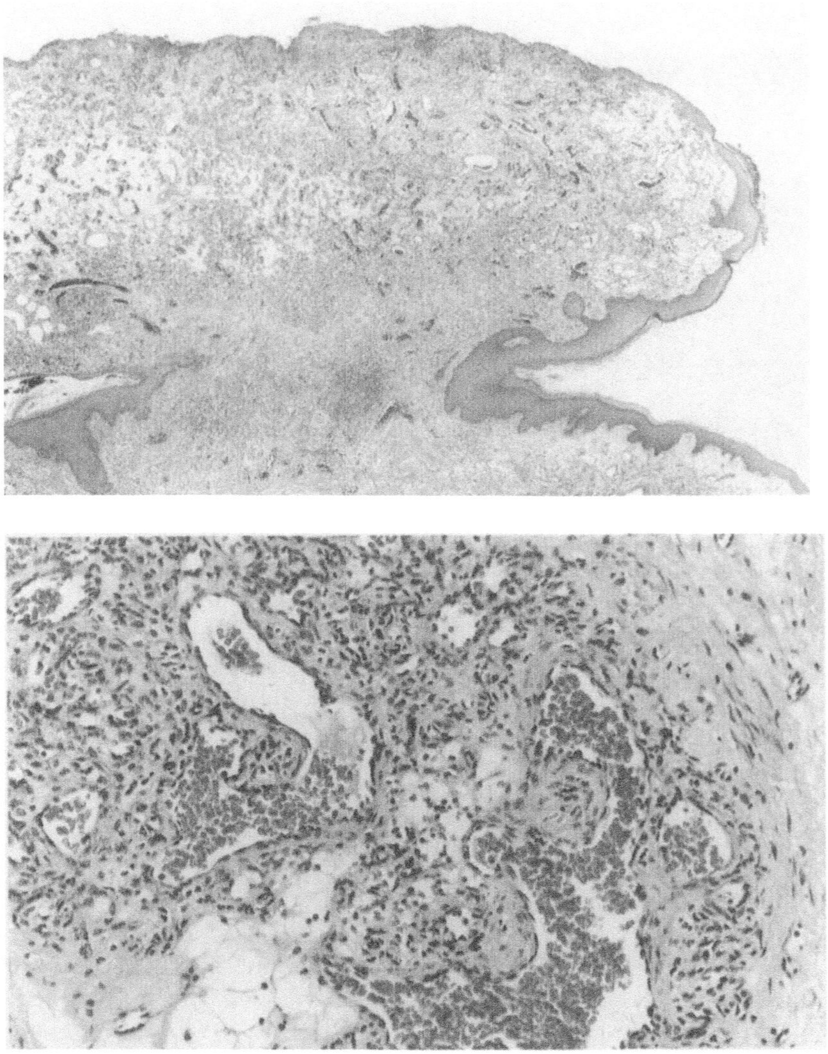

a b

Fig. 122a,b. *Pyogenic granuloma.* **a** An ulcerated, polypoid lesion with a collarette of epidermis. **b** Thin-walled blood vessels of varied size embedded in oedematous, inflamed stroma

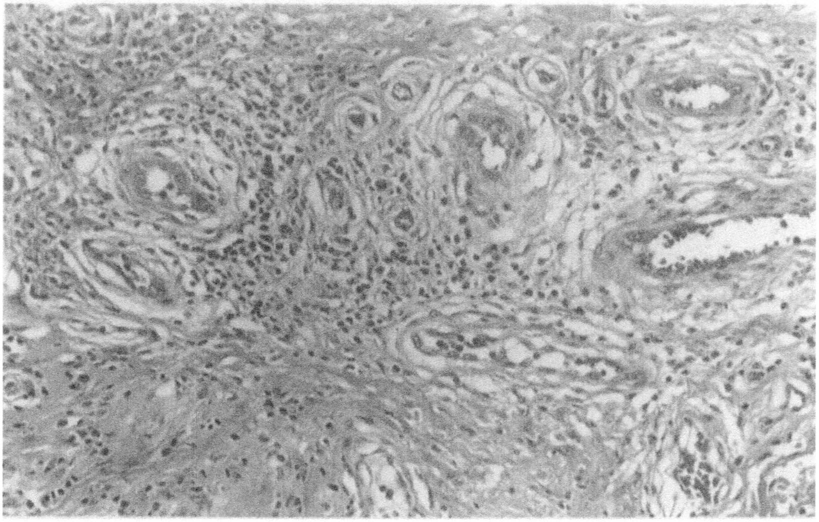

Fig. 123. *Angiolymphoid hyperplasia with eosinophilia (epithelioid haemangioma).* Small blood vessels lined by plump epithelioid endothelial cells, with a lymphohistiocytic infiltrate and scattered eosinophils in the stroma

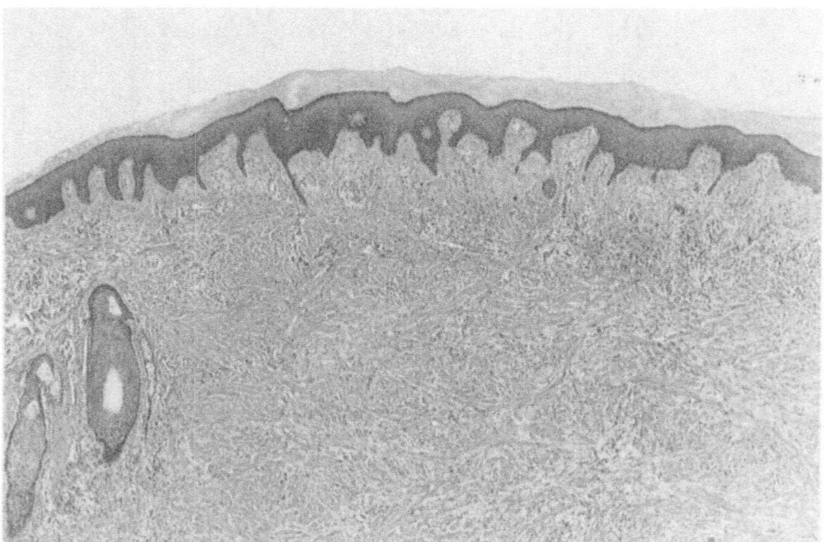

Fig. 124a. *Benign fibrous histiocytoma.* The epidermis is hyperplastic and separated by a grenz zone from a diffusely cellular tumour in the dermis

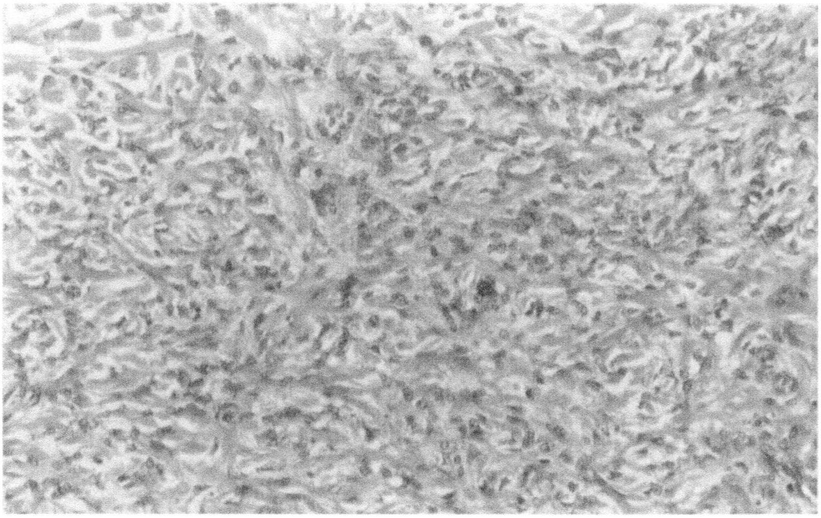

Fig. 124b. *Benign fibrous histiocytoma.* The neoplasm is composed of plump spindle cells and histiocytes in a collagenous stroma

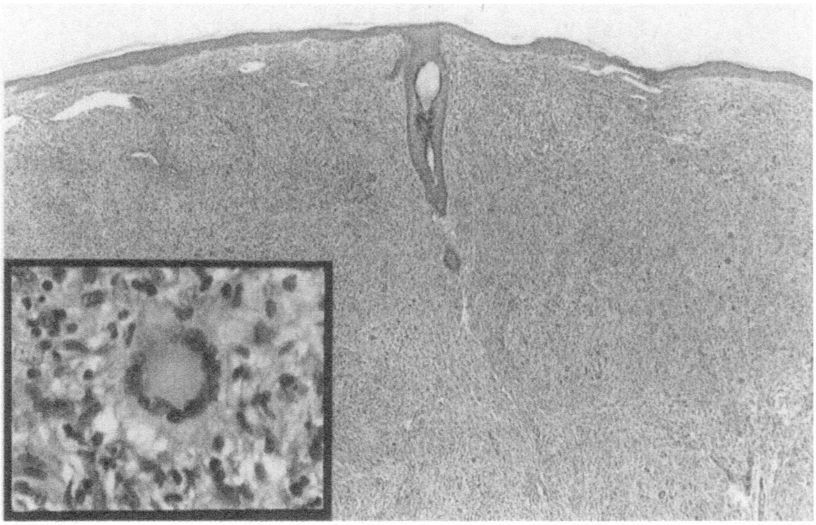

Fig. 125. *Benign (juvenile) xanthogranuloma.* A diffuse infiltrate extending into the deep dermis. *Inset*, spindle cells, lymphocytes and a central Touton giant cell

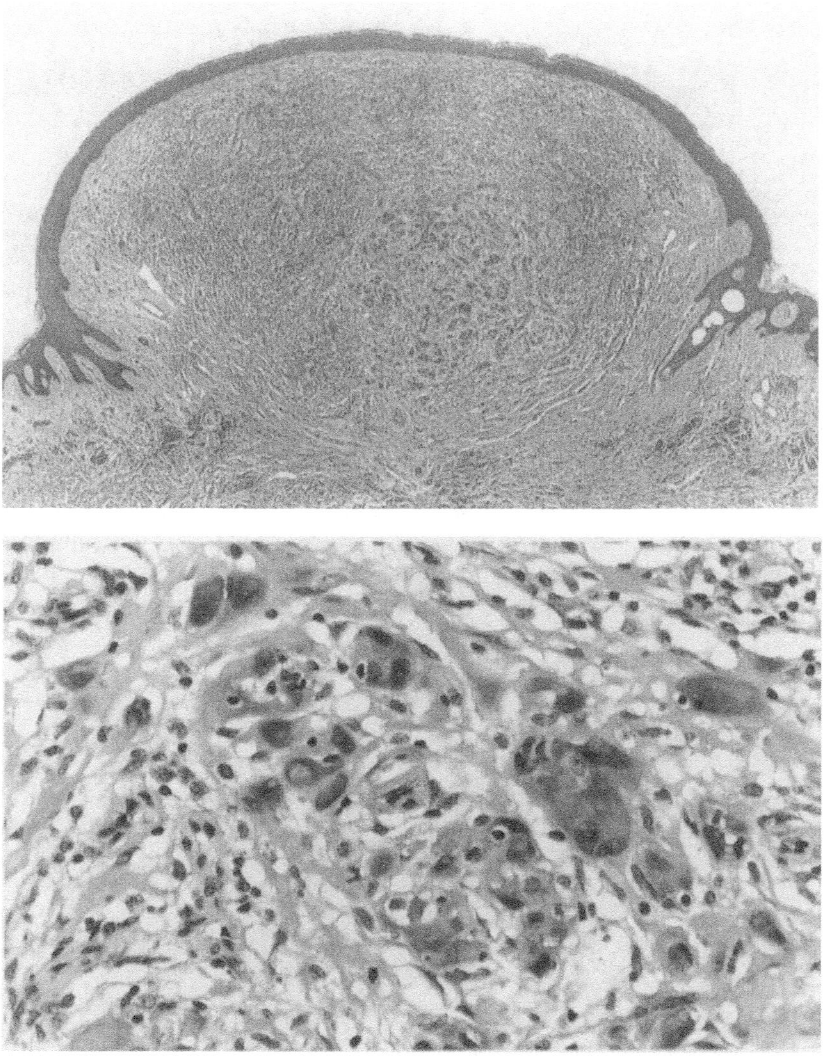

a

b

Fig. 126a,b. *Reticulohistiocytoma.* **a** A dome-shaped nodular lesion composed of a dermal infiltrate of spindle cells and giant cells. **b** Macrophages, giant cells and lymphocytes in a collagenous stroma

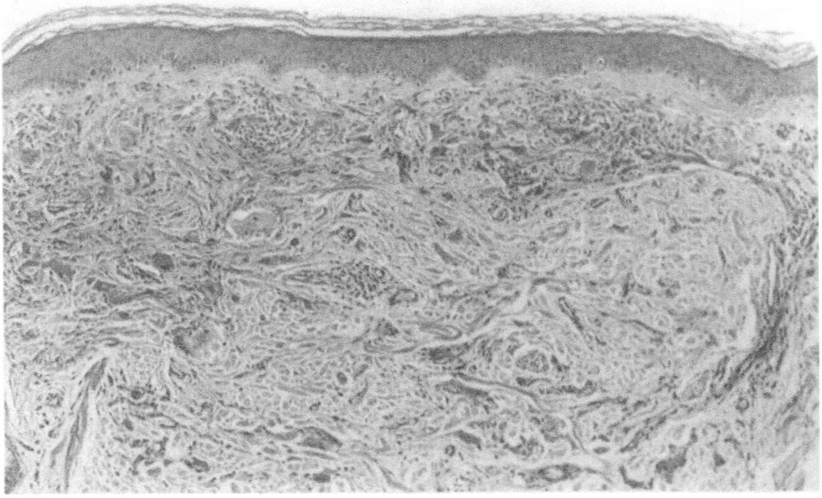

a

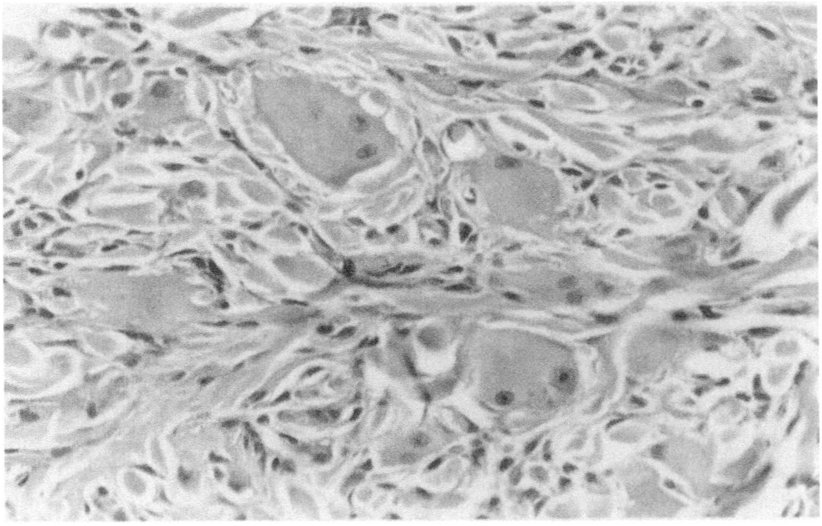

b

Fig. 127a,b. *Multicentric reticulohistiocytosis.* **a** Giant cells arranged singly in the upper dermis. **b** Multinucleated giant cells with ground-glass cytoplasm

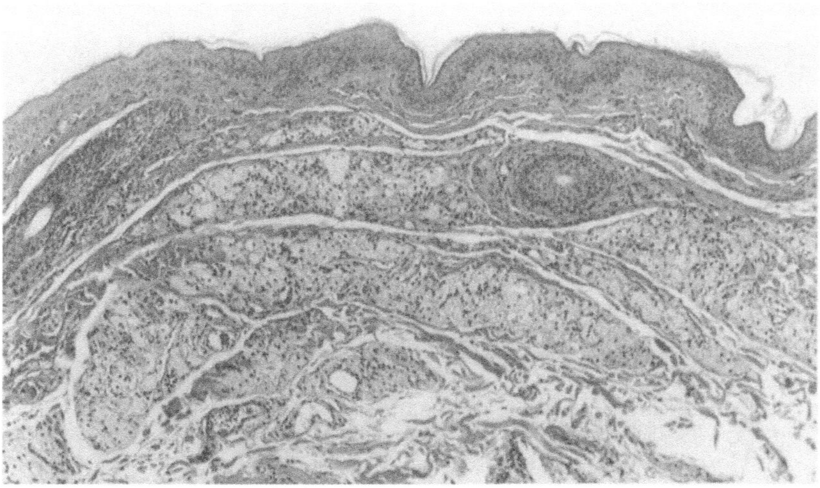

Fig. 128. *Xanthoma.* Groups of lipid-laden macrophages in the superficial and deep dermis

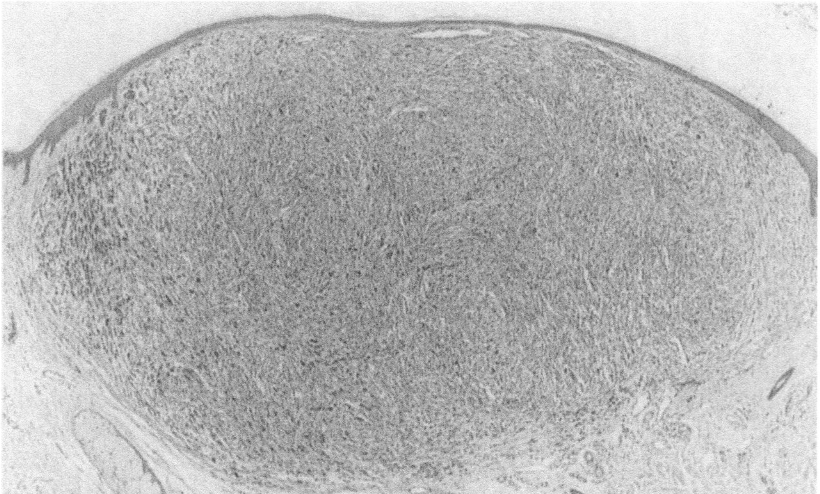

Fig. 129a. *Atypical fibroxanthoma.* A circumscribed nodular mass of pleomorphic spindle cells elevates the epidermis and extends into the deep dermis

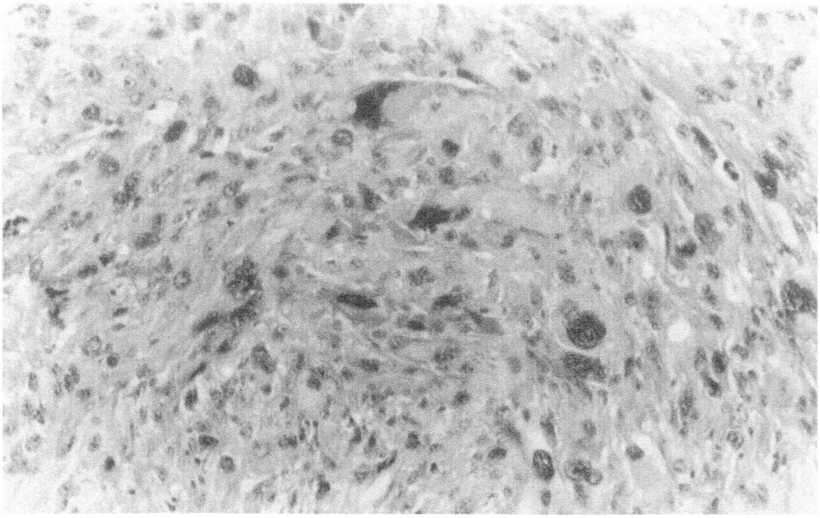

Fig. 129b. *Atypical fibroxanthoma.* Pleomorphic spindle cells and giant cells with bizarre, hyperchromatic nuclei

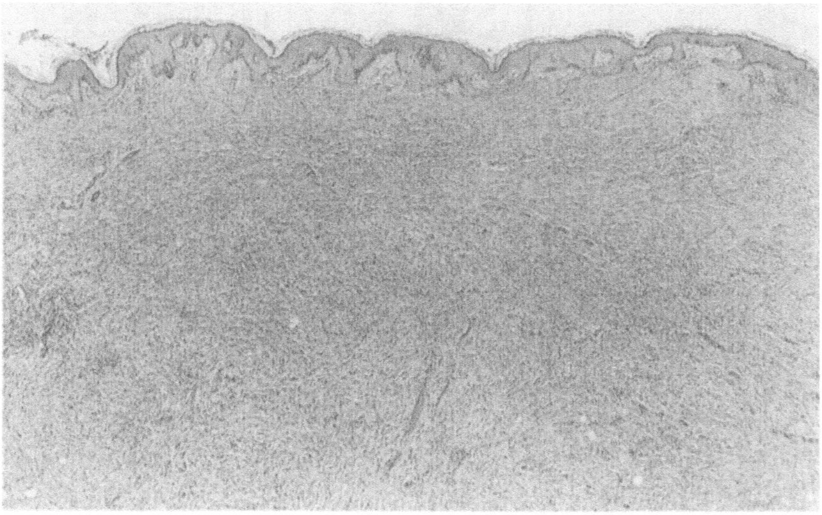

Fig. 130a. *Dermatofibrosarcoma protuberans.* Dense proliferation of spindle cells in diffuse pattern throughout the dermis

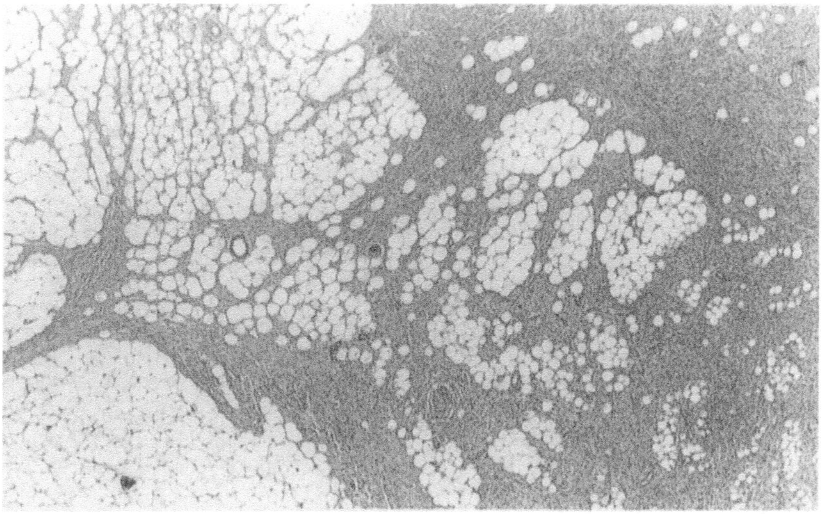
b

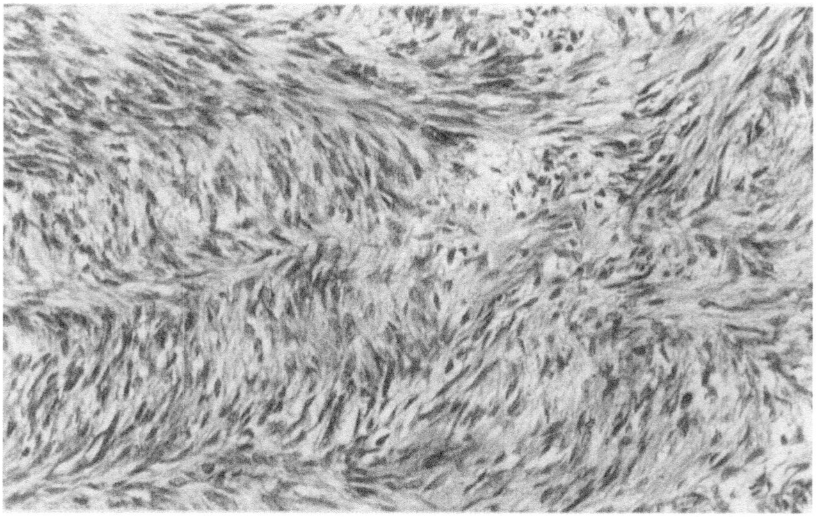
c

Fig. 130b,c. *Dermatofibrosarcoma protuberans.* **b** Infiltration of subcutaneous fat by broad trabeculae and slender strands of neoplastic spindle cells, producing a honeycomb pattern. **c** Prominent storiform pattern

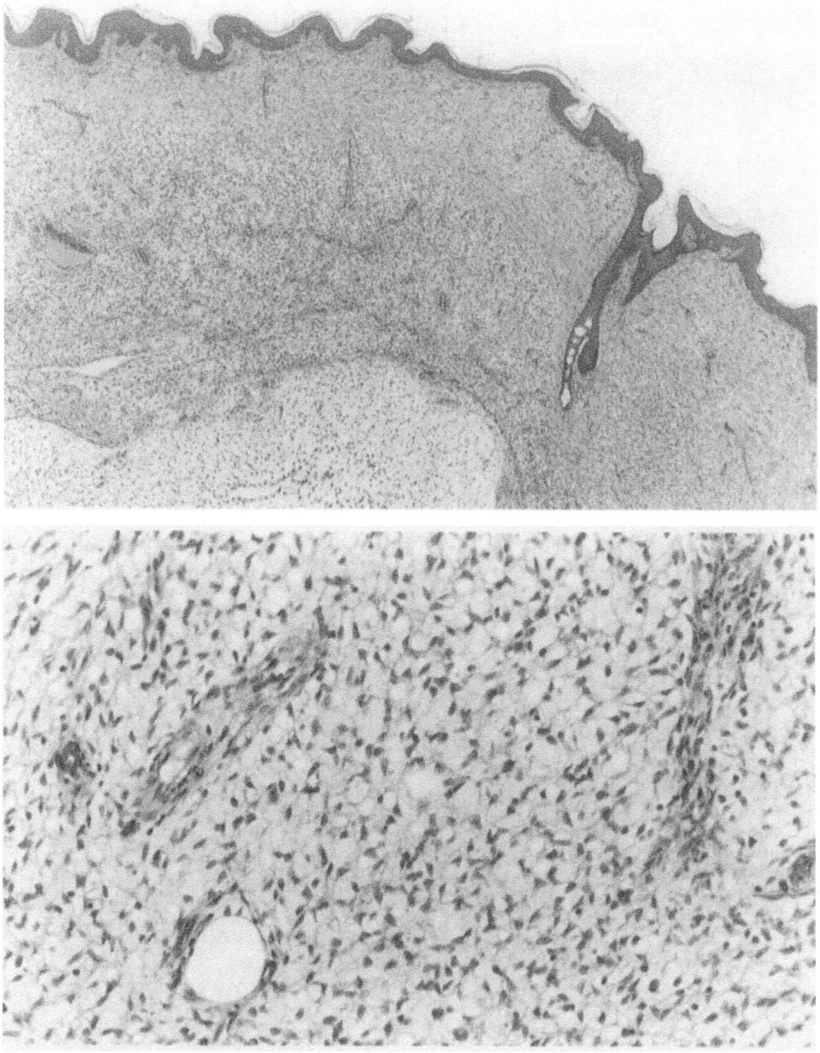
d
e

Fig. 130d,e. *Dermatofibrosarcoma protuberans.* **d** Myxoid dermatofibrosarcoma protuberans. Myxoid nodular component in the deep dermis. **e** The spindle cells are separated by pale-staining connective tissue mucin

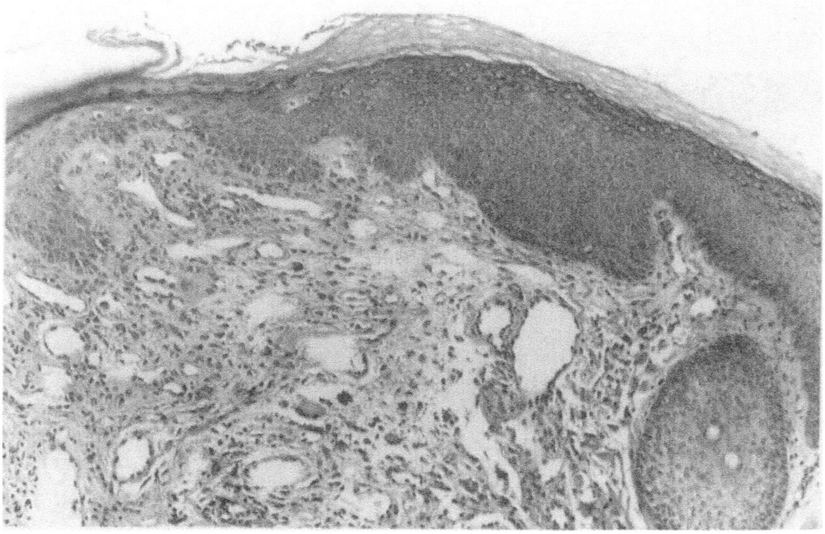

Fig. 131. *Adenoma sebaceum.* Dermal angiofibromatous proliferation with spindle cells and giant cells in the stroma

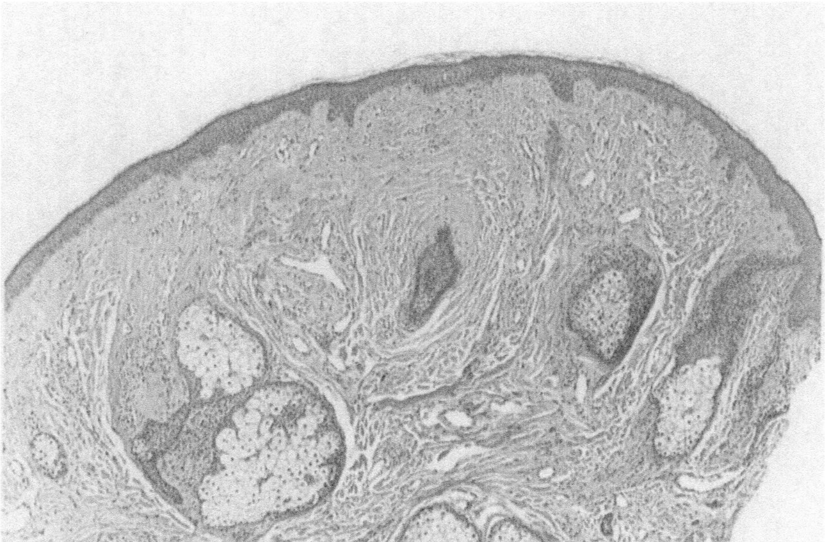

Fig. 132. *Fibrous papule.* The epidermis is raised overlying a zone of vascular fibroplasia with scattered spindle cells in the superficial dermis

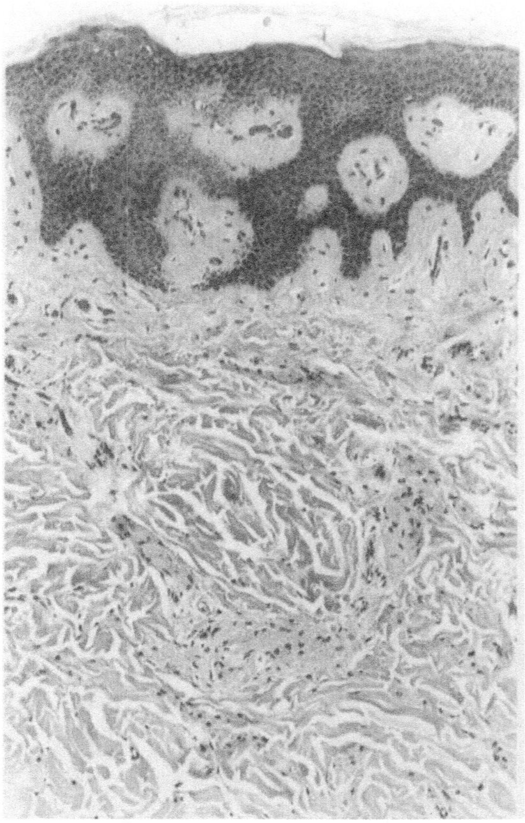

a

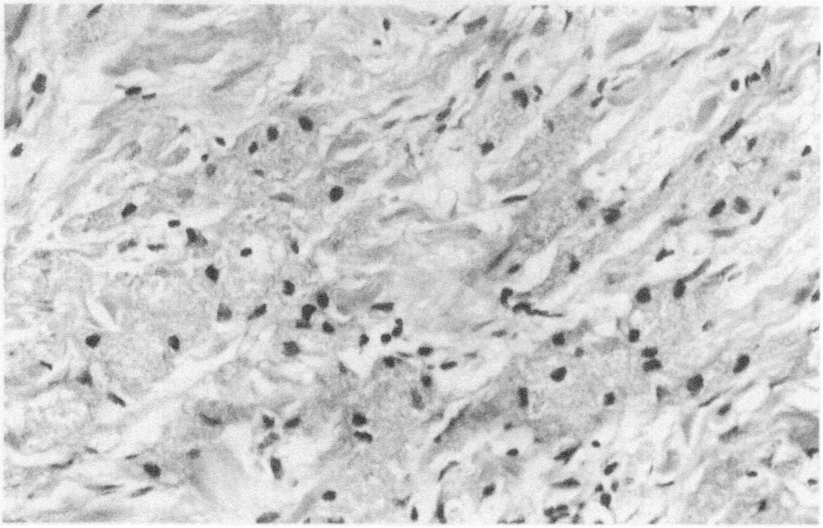

b

Fig. 133a,b. *Granular cell tumour.* **a** Hyperplastic epidermis overlies strands and groups of cells with abundant eosinophilic cytoplasm and small nuclei. **b** The neoplastic cells have coarsely granular cytoplasm and small hyperchromatic nuclei

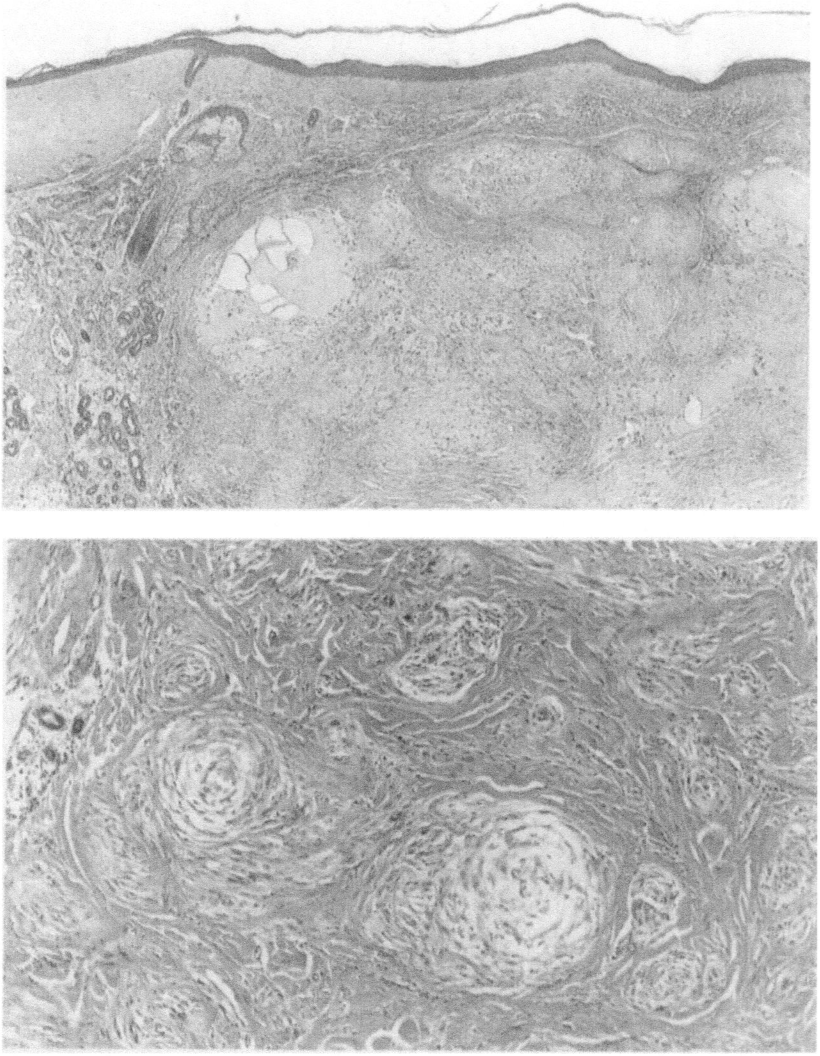

a

b

Fig. 134a,b. *Neurothekeoma.* **a** Circumscribed lobules including myxoid areas. **b** Whorls of spindle cells and collagen surround small myxoid areas

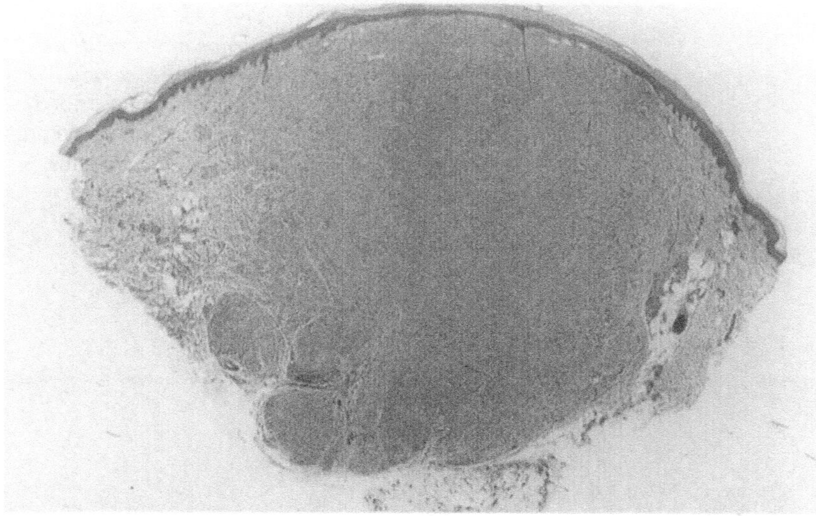

a

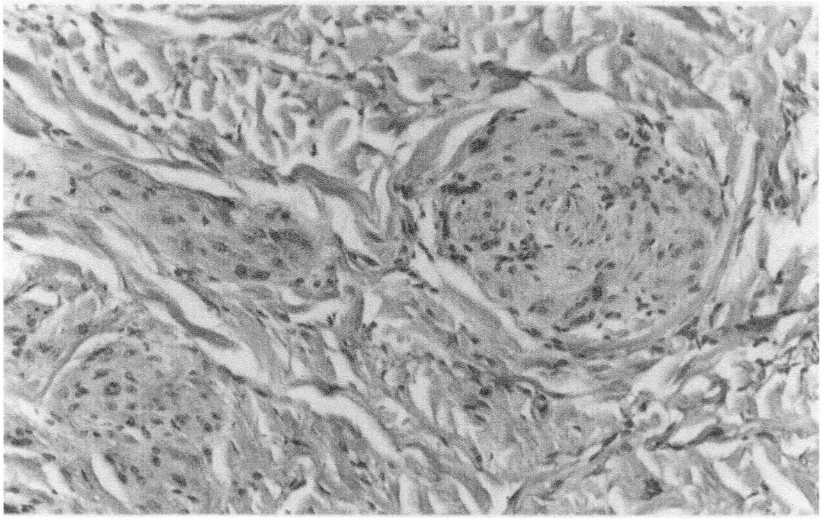

b

Fig. 135a,b. *Cellular neurothekeoma.* **a** Well-defined, densely cellular, multilobular tumour in the dermis and subcutis. **b** Plump spindle cells in small groups (*left*) and surrounding a nerve (*right*)

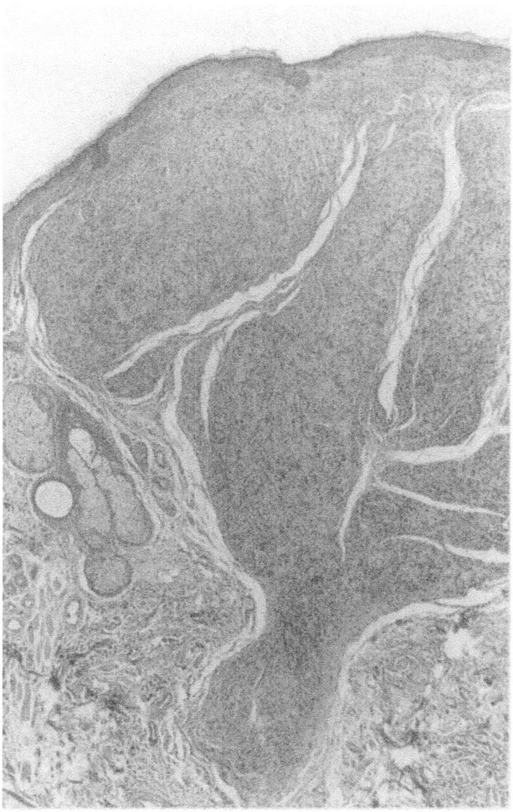

Fig. 136. *Palisaded encapsulated neuroma (solitary neuroma).* Sharply circumscribed, cellular nodules extending into the deep dermis

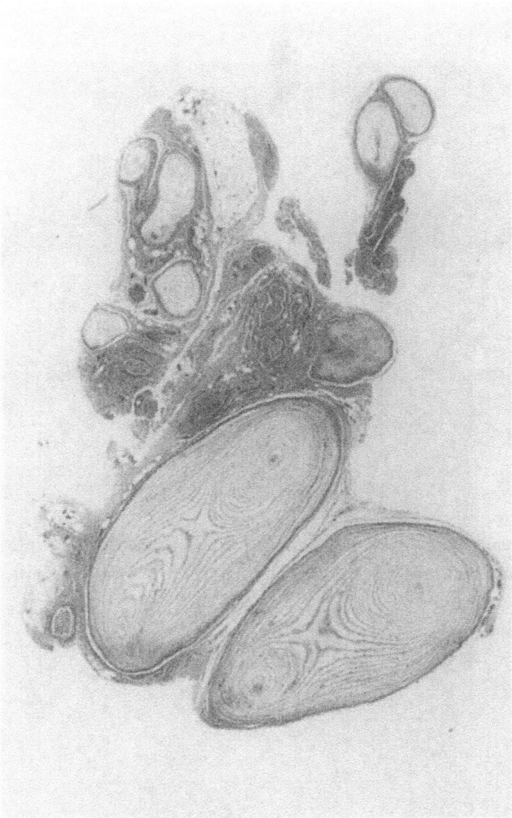

Fig. 137. *Pacinian neurofibroma (pacinioma).* Large ovoid, corpuscular, lamellated structures

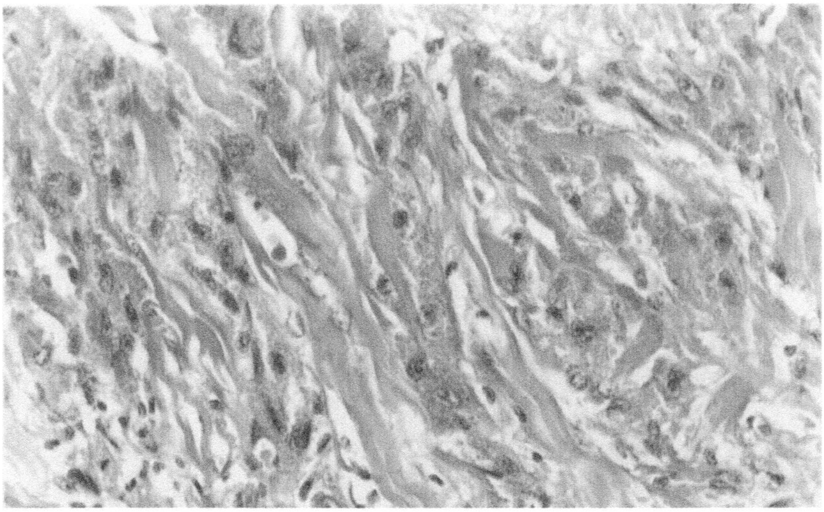

Fig. 138. *Malignant granular cell tumour.* The neoplastic cells have abundant, coarsely granular cytoplasm and moderately pleomorphic nuclei. This tumour metastasized

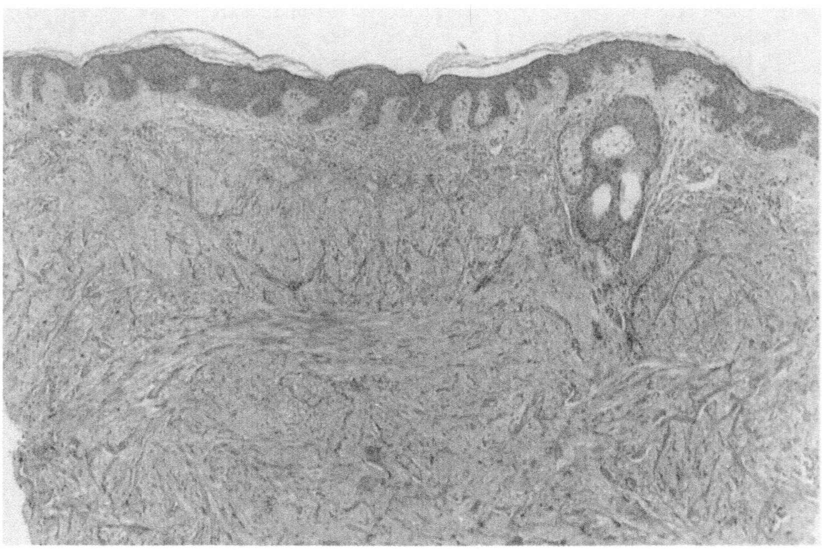

Fig. 139a. *Piloleiomyoma.* Interlocking bundles of smooth muscle in the dermis, separated from the epidermis by a clear zone

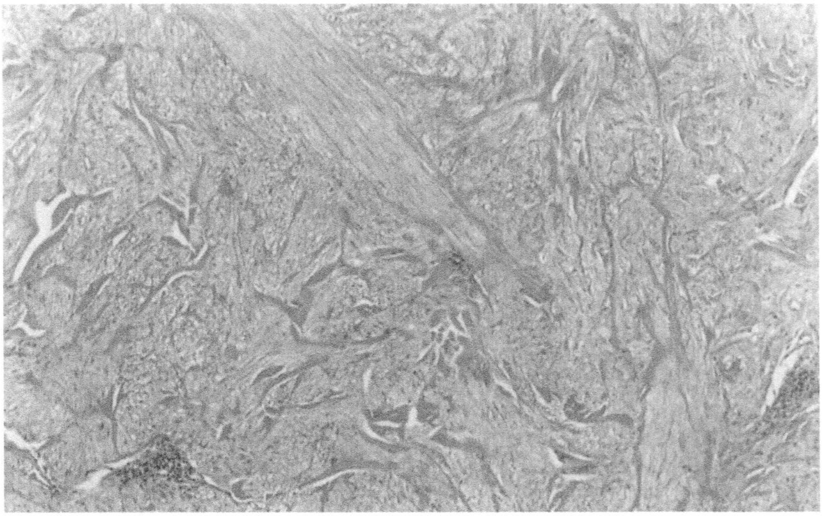

Fig. 139b. *Piloleiomyoma.* Bundles of muscle surround a segment of arrector pili

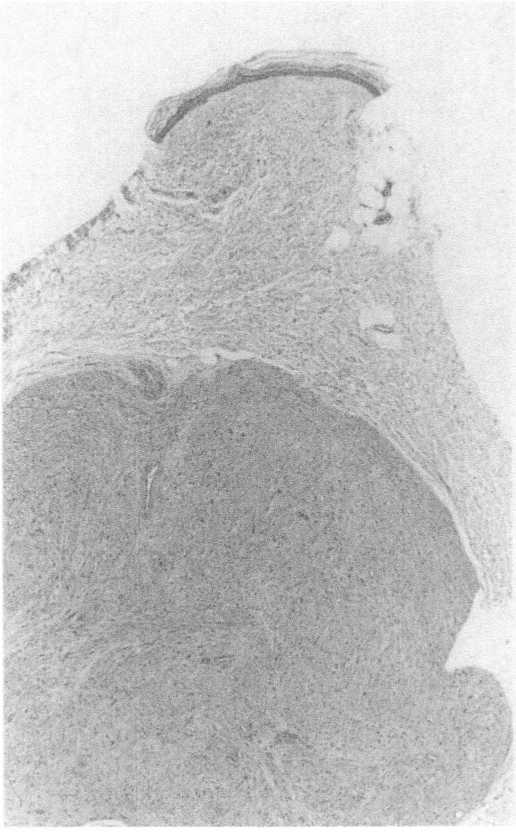

Fig. 140a. *Angioleiomyoma.* Circumscribed, densely cellular nodules in the deep dermis

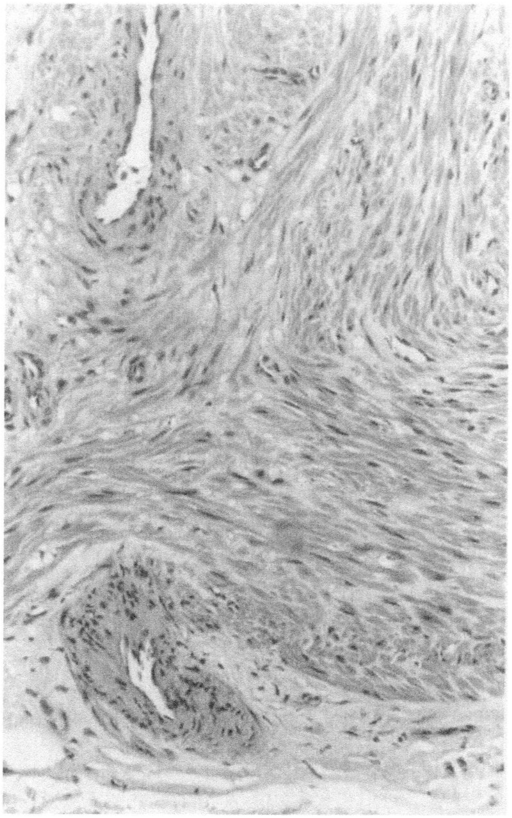

Fig. 140b. *Angioleiomyoma.* Uniform smooth muscle cells in interlocking strands surrounding and merging with the walls of blood vessels

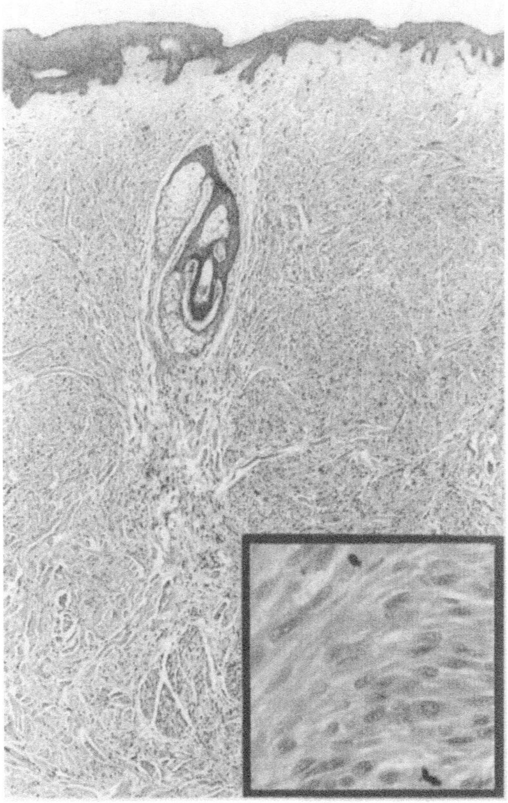

Fig. 141. *Superficial leiomyosarcoma.* Dermal invasion by interlocking fascicles of smooth muscle cells. *Inset*, the neoplastic cells have blunt-ended, moderately pleomorphic nuclei with numerous mitoses

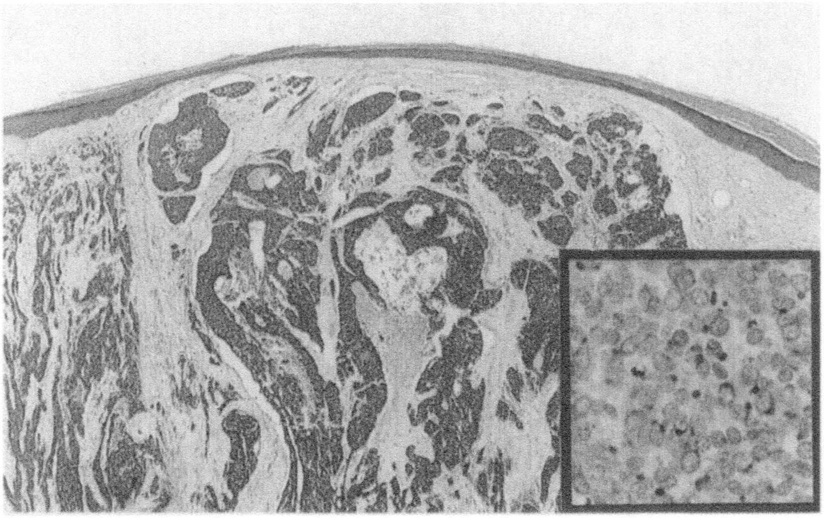

Fig. 142a. *Primary cutaneous neuroendocrine carcinoma (Merkel cell tumour).* A low-power view of neuroendocrine carcinoma infiltrating the dermis in trabecular and nodular patterns. *Inset*, positive immunostaining for CAM5.2 cytokeratin, showing the typical paranuclear globular pattern

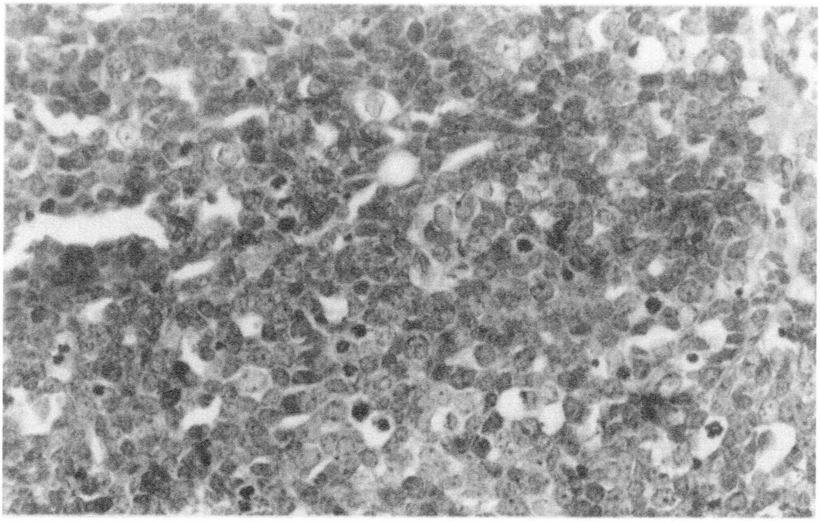

Fig. 142b. *Primary cutaneous neuroendocrine carcinoma (Merkel cell tumour).* Dense sheets of neuroendocrine cells with scanty cytoplasm, granular chromatin and single cell necrosis

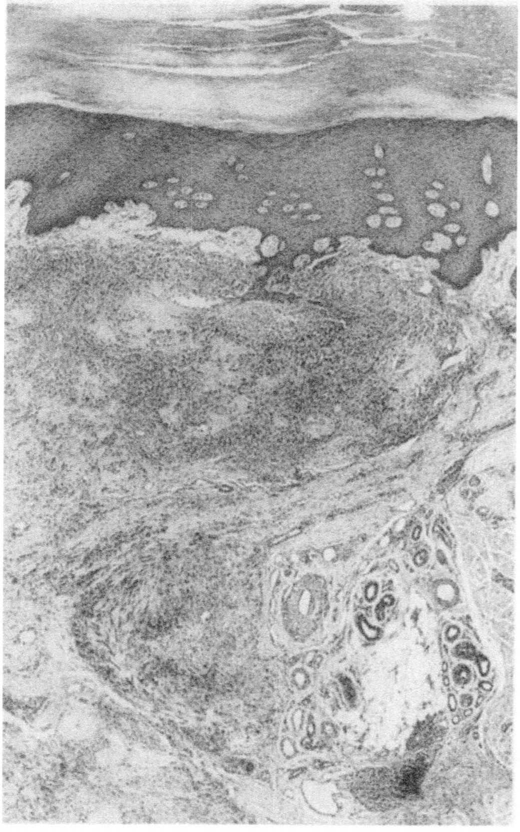

Fig. 143a. *Epithelioid sarcoma.* Ill-defined nodules and zones of necrosis extending into the deep dermis

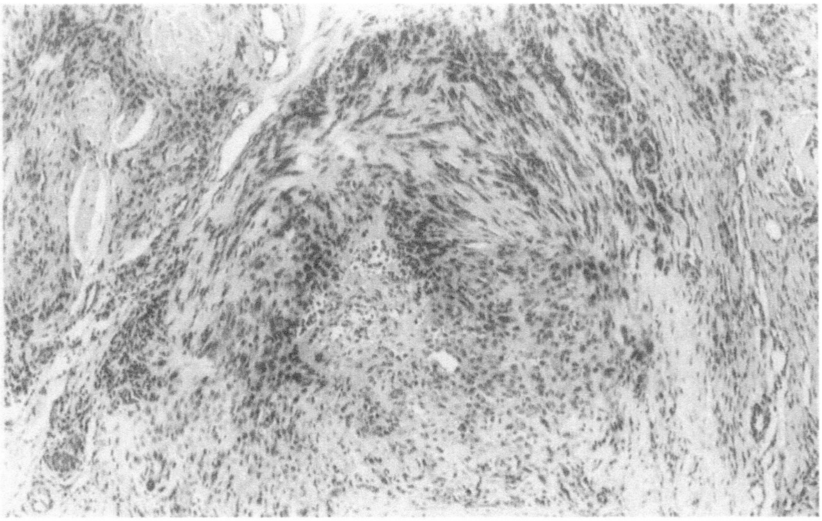

b

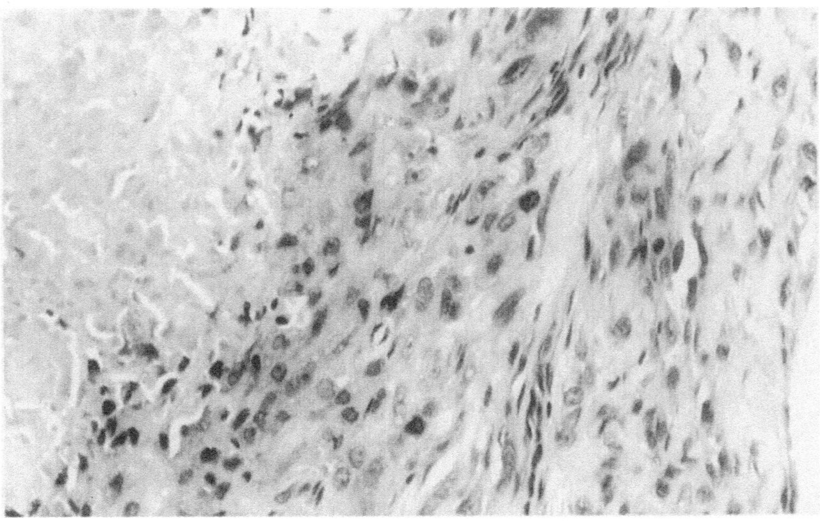

c

Fig. 143b,c. *Epithelioid sarcoma.* **b** Nodules of epithelioid and spindle cells with central foci of necrosis. **c** Necrosis (*left*) in a nodule of spindle and epithelioid cells with pleomorphic, hyperchromatic nuclei

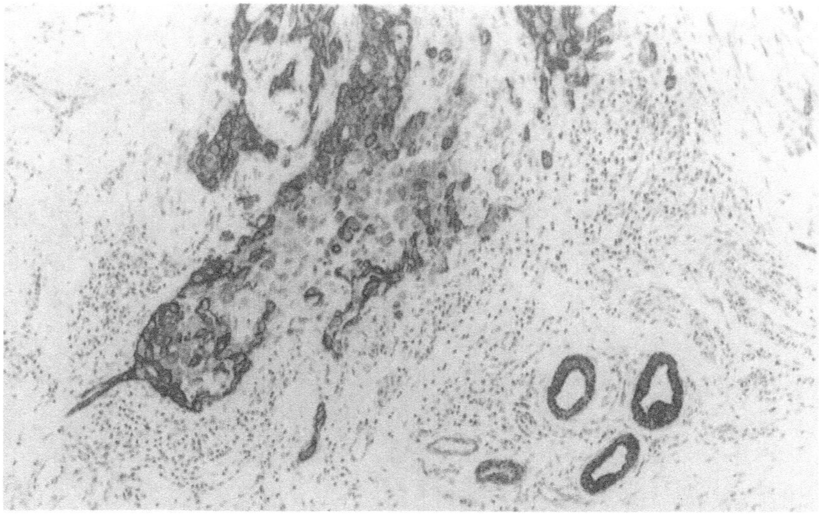

Fig. 143d. *Epithelioid sarcoma.* Positive immunostaining for cytokeratin CAM5.2 in the neoplastic cells

Subject Index

Springer-Verlag and the Environment

We at Springer-Verlag firmly believe that an international science publisher has a special obligation to the environment, and our corporate policies consistently reflect this conviction.

We also expect our business partners – paper mills, printers, packaging manufacturers, etc. – to commit themselves to using environmentally friendly materials and production processes.

The paper in this book is made from low- or no-chlorine pulp and is acid free, in conformance with international standards for paper permanency.

GPSR Compliance

The European Union's (EU) General Product Safety Regulation (GPSR) is a set of rules that requires consumer products to be safe and our obligations to ensure this.

If you have any concerns about our products, you can contact us on ProductSafety@springernature.com

In case Publisher is established outside the EU, the EU authorized representative is:

Springer Nature Customer Service Center GmbH
Europaplatz 3
69115 Heidelberg, Germany

Batch number: 10704771

Printed by Printforce, the Netherlands